WITH A
FOREWORD BY
#1 *New York Times*
bestselling author
JOY
BAUER

Give PEAS a Chance

The foolproof guide to feeding your picky toddler

Kate Samela

MS, RD, CSP

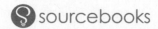

sourcebooks

Published by Sourcebooks, Inc.
P.O. Box 4410, Naperville, Illinois 60567-4410
(630) 961-3900
Fax: (630) 961-2168
www.sourcebooks.com

Library of Congress Cataloging-in-Publication Data

Samela, Kate.
  Give peas a chance : the foolproof guide to feeding your picky toddler / Kate Samela, MS, RD, CSP.
      pages cm
  (pbk. : alk. paper) 1. Toddlers--Nutrition. I. Title.
  RJ216.S367 2012
  649'.3--dc23

                                    2012031246

Printed and bound in the United States of America.
VP 10 9 8 7 6 5 4 3 2 1

Dedication

For my mother, Patsy...for everything.

Contents

Foreword

I first met Kate in 2003. I was the founder and CEO of one of the largest nutrition centers in the country, and we were in need of a topnotch pediatric specialist. My clientele expected the best. After an extensive hunt and countless interviews, all roads led to Kate Samela. I was elated when she agreed to join my prestigious team in New York City, and it took all of five minutes for Kate to make an impressive name for herself among patients, as well as referring physicians. You're in good hands with Kate—she's the rock star of pediatric nutrition. Kate is a superstar mom and a down-to-earth, strategic dietitian I feel lucky to have as a friend and colleague.

But full disclosure: I don't like peas!

I'm willing to bet that if you've picked up this book, you're probably a parent or soon-to-be-parent who is concerned about your child's overall health. That means you deserve kudos right off the bat. You've recognized how important it is to set your child up with good eating habits at a young age. Plus, the best weapon against obesity is a healthy relationship with food, and your support is invaluable in helping your children start that relationship well.

If you've wandered onto these pages because meals have become a time of frustration, coaxing, pleading, or tears, I want to start by offering you three simple words of comfort: *you're not alone*. While each child's food preferences are different, kids do have one thing in common: almost every little guy or gal has food issues at one age or another. Believe me, my own kids are a work in progress. My oldest daughter Jesse went through an anticalcium phase, and my youngest, Ayden, has a raging sweet tooth I occasionally need to tame. Don't blame yourself for your child's reluctance to eat broccoli or try a chopped apple. Toddlers are hard-wired to be suspicious of new flavors and often forget to eat because they are so busy exploring the world around them. While it may not always be a pleasant or easy experience (ahem!) trying to get your child to eat, it is completely normal. And your hard work will pay off in the end. While you may need to offer a certain food to your child several times before he becomes comfortable with it, odds are pretty darn good that he will eventually accept it—and maybe even learn to love it. And if he never comes around to a particular food, that's okay, too—there are still plenty of opportunities to ensure your child gets the nutrition he or she needs, sans spinach, quinoa, tofu…and yes, um, even peas.

This book can give you the tools to do just that. *Give Peas a Chance* provides practical, parent-tested advice for moms, dads, and caretakers of picky eaters. Kate's thirteen years as a nutritionist, as well as her invaluable experience as a mother of two terrific kids, give her both the professional and personal know-how to provide smart, realistic strategies that make a difference at mealtime. With Kate's creative, flexible approach, and a little trial and error at the kitchen table, I am confident that you will discover which foods and strategies work best for you and your family.

Yes, good nutrition is important, especially in early childhood. *Yes*, you want your child to develop a healthy rapport with food. But at the same time, try your best to keep the whole "food thing" in perspective and look at the big picture, rather than getting stressed about every mealtime hiccup. If your daughter eats all her broccoli one night and outright refuses it the next, it's not cause for alarm—in fact, it is completely normal behavior, especially for the ever-evolving toddler. As you'll learn in the pages that follow, your reaction to your child's behavior will have a much greater impact on her long-term relationship with food than anything three stalks of broccoli can contribute to her health at that moment.

I can't recommend this book enough. Kate has compiled all of her experience and research on the terrors of feeding toddlers into an indispensable, no-nonsense guide, and the result will help any frustrated family bring some peace back to the dinner table. Happy reading and feeding!

—Joy Bauer, nutrition expert
and bestselling author of *Joy's LIFE Diet*

Introduction

As I sit here and think about what happened tonight at my very own dinner table, I burst out laughing at the thought that *I* am the person writing this book, a book specifically about how to introduce new foods to picky toddlers; a book that unravels toddler development and essentially explains to parents why almost every toddler is hardwired to be "picky"; a book that urges frantic parents to keep calm, cool, and collected at all times in regard to feeding—despite how much food your tot actually swallows; a book that *in essence* reminds you that feeding is not perfect—and that it's OK to have the meals that are, well, less than perfect. All I can say is that I am glad our dinnertime tonight was not broadcast on YouTube for the world of potential readers to view as both my son Jake, now seven, and my daughter Maggie, just four, looked at me in utter disbelief that I made ravioli—with something other than cheese on the inside.

At first mortified at the thought of someone witnessing this scene, I quickly stopped to wonder—what if dinnertime at my house was on YouTube tonight? Could it be a good thing?

Watching me, mother first, pediatric dietitian last, fall into coaxing both of my children to "just take a bite" and try this Martian ravioli. (For the record, it was pesto, and it seemed like a good thing to buy at the time.)

Watching my son Jake spit out his pesto ravioli—properly on a napkin, thank you very much—moaning in sheer despair as his taste buds registered "unfamiliar flavor: get it out!" (I prayed the neighbors were all inside as he carried on like a wounded animal on prime time Discovery. I mean really, I can't help but wonder what would have happened if they were portobello-stuffed...)

Laughing all the while as my daughter Maggie, surprisingly very willing to try new foods, takes a bite, scrapes it off her tongue, and declares, "These are disgusting!"

And could it really be a good thing, considering the preacher of family dinners is missing a very important someone at the dinner table (scandalous!) on this particular night, that someone being Dad?

So far, this YouTube possibility seems like a bad idea—maybe even awful.

BUT WHAT IF I ASKED IF YOU NOTICED...

...How the coaxing was short-lived, as I pulled my professional self together and tried desperately to remain neutral for the rest of dinner by eloquently redirecting conversation about what went on during the day.

...How Jake went about the meal and declared he was going to eat only his broccoli, meatballs, and garlic bread on his plate—but not *those ravioli*. Fine by me, I thought quietly in my head, resisting my desire to applaud his decision.

...How Maggie, following in her older brother's footsteps, chose to eat the part of her meal she liked as well: one and a half small meatballs, equal to a ping pong ball, giving her just about all the protein she needed for the whole day, with three small trees of broccoli (check one serving of veggie), and the squishy inside of three thinly sliced pieces of garlic bread (check carbohydrate). All washed down with about a quarter cup of 1% organic milk.

AND YOU MIGHT NOT HAVE SEEN...

The three of us shuffling out to the car and racing toward hockey practice, where we find Jake's coach, Dad, anxiously waiting to lace up his skates in locker room number three.

Though it was a bit hectic, I hope you can see the small successes of that particular meal—because we all know the outcome could have been a lot worse. For me, my goals were met. I felt good about what my kids ate, how much they ate, how they were sitting down to eat, and most importantly, how we got to spend that twenty minutes (OK, maybe fifteen) sitting at the table—together.

Even though I am a registered dietitian, just like you I am constantly in search of the perfect balance between the dos and the don'ts of feeding a family—especially the ever-challenging toddler. *Give Peas a Chance* will give you the tools to feel good about what and how much your toddler is eating and allow you to enjoy mealtimes together—minus the stress.

WHY WRITE A BOOK SPECIFICALLY ABOUT TODDLER NUTRITION?

As a registered dietitian (RD) and a specialist in pediatric nutrition, I take care of infants and children throughout all stages of the life cycle. Toddlers, who will be defined for the purposes of this book as ages one to three years, are some of the most vivacious yet demanding creatures on Earth. One minute they're your friend; in a nanosecond, they're your enemy—often for what appears to be no good reason at all. It has taken me twelve years of working in this field and having two children to understand that feeding a toddler is ten percent about actual food and nutrition and ninety percent about parenting. Through my work and home life, I have come to fully understand that feeding a toddler and parenting go hand in hand, and I am excited to share some of the secrets I have learned about toddlers that will make feeding during this life stage more enjoyable—for everyone.

Having been fortunate enough to work with hundreds of families at some of the preeminent pediatric hospitals in the nation, I have developed a tremendous understanding of what makes children grow—even under the direst of circumstances. At the beginning of my career, I worked with undernourished, critically ill children where I saw firsthand what a task it was for them to eat. I was committed to making it easier for sick children to gain or sustain their body weight. I counted endless calories and grams of protein and trained myself to write prescriptions for how much food was enough. Once my career path changed and I began to work with young children who were not critically ill, a specific population of "troubled eaters" quickly surfaced with each consultation. Most were toddlers who were simply driving their parents mad with each and every bite of food (or lack thereof!). I soon realized that the one- to three-year-olds I saw for "feeding difficulties" typically fell into one of the following four categories.

1. Grazers

Toddlers who were offered food, milk, or juice whenever they asked for it because

a) their parents had been told that their tot's weight was faltering a bit from the growth curve;

OR

b) parental perception of how much food their toddler *should* be eating versus how much the toddler actually ate.

Well-intended parents were often more exhausted from trying to get their toddler to eat than from the toddler himself. In many cases, parents were confessing to me that they were leaving random snacks around the house (e.g., Goldfish crackers on the coffee table, the remainder of breakfast on the table right up until lunchtime) and toting snacks just about everywhere in case the toddler got hungry. After taking countless diet histories from families and listening to endless feeding schedules, it became evident that the grazers were able to eat just enough food every one to two hours to squelch their hunger cues and keep their blood sugar in check, but never really had the chance to develop physical hunger to eat enough food at mealtimes. So, when breakfast, lunch, or dinner rolled around, there was zero motivation to come sit down and eat, and if the toddler *did* make an attempt to eat (usually after a battle of wills), only a few bites of food were consumed. The result? Parents felt that their toddlers "ate nothing!"

> *Secret #1: Toddlers need very small amounts of food to grow and thrive. After the first year of life, their growth rapidly slows down and their calorie needs decrease. From birth to one year of age, an infant will essentially triple his or her birth weight. A toddler's rate of growth is much slower. A two-year-old may gain only four pounds by the time he or she is three, which is only about 15 percent of his or her body weight.*

2. Excess Empty-Calorie Consumers

It has become increasingly clear that in today's very hectic lifestyle, parents are frustrated with their toddler's ability to eat foods from the family table. So many families neglect cooking meals for a lot of reasons: lack of interest, time, and patience, particularly with young toddlers in the home; when effort is put into cooking and the toddler doesn't eat, the line seems to be drawn—in concrete. So many parents come into the office starting the conversation with the same sentence: "He just won't eat what we eat." When probed, the story would go something like this: "He only ate a few bites of baked chicken and maybe a few spoonfuls of carrots, so I made him a hot dog." As time went on, I came to understand that parents feel compelled to feed their toddler "something" at every meal, so they resort to feeding junk or snack-type foods if the toddler doesn't appear to eat enough table food, or what I like to refer to in this book as **proper food**.

Secret #2: Toddler development is unique when it comes to feeding and food choices. Let's think about the first six months of an infant's life: she is essentially on a liquid diet; she eats, sleeps, and poops; developmentally, she is working on trust and is relatively immobile. For the most part, she can be contained in a high chair and is willing to consume what she is given. When she reaches toddlerhood, she is learning to talk and walk, which means she is able to say no with authority and can hop down from the table at any given moment (if allowed), not to mention working tirelessly at learning to feed herself. This new person can't help but offer her opinion when she has the chance and takes every opportunity to express how she feels—simply because she can. This is quite a change from the relative ease of feeding a snuggly baby around the clock every three to four hours in response to a simple cry. Couple this with the transition from jarred baby food in perfectly portioned containers labeled with calories, and it is crystal clear that parents feel disarmed when it comes to quantifying how much table food is, in fact, enough.

3. Excessive Drinkers

Toddlers who come into my office with a nine-ounce sippy cup in tow are some of the most frequent flyers I see for what doctors refer to as "poor weight gain." These toddlers were either taking in large quantities of milk with very little table food, causing some to develop outright anemia, or had stopped taking milk altogether and had begun consuming large amounts of juice with a limited variety of foods. In either circumstance, weight gain was less than ideal, and appetites were minimal. In addition, the toddlers who were drinking excess juice were experiencing diarrhea, which was another frustration for parents during potty training and definitely did not help with weight gain.

> Secret #3: Toddlers should not be drinking more than thirty-two ounces of liquid per day. Liquids fill up a toddler's little tummy as it is about the size of a tennis ball to a baseball. Ideally, a toddler will take sixteen to twenty-four ounces of milk per day, with the remaining eight ounces as a combination of water and 100% fruit juice.

4. Fat-Free Consumers

As the headlines remind us of how unhealthy American eating habits have become, many families have embraced the dietary guidelines from the American

Dietetic Association, the American Heart Association, and the National Cancer Institute, which all recommend a low-fat or non-fat diet. Unfortunately these guidelines, which can be healthy for many school-age kids, adolescents, and adults, present a problem for the young toddler who is eating what his parents eat at the family table. I see a surprising number of families who, in an effort to follow a healthy diet, actually are unintentionally depriving their toddlers of the fat in food their growing bodies and brains desperately need.

> *Secret #4: A fundamental association between dietary patterns and human health has been overlooked since the dawn of the low-fat diet: the essential need for dietary fat. Despite the increasing epidemic of obese children we are reminded about in the media daily, our toddlers need to have up to 40 percent of their calories from fat in order to support both body and brain growth. More importantly, fat plays a critical role in how food tastes, and promotes a sense of fullness after eating—one of our biggest defenses against the war on obesity.*

The confusion surrounding feeding toddlers became more obvious with each family I met. Evidently, something that seemed so basic and innate in raising a child had become a daunting task for many parents. Time and time again, I found myself giving the same advice and reassurance to families if their toddlers fell into one of the above categories. *Give Peas a Chance* will help you gain an understanding of how a toddler grows, how much food a toddler needs to grow, and how to approach feeding a toddler. This book will help you take stock and identify where you might be in your own battle. Even if you are simply seeking reassurance that your toddler is on track and properly nourished, you will have the opportunity to connect the dots between your toddler's nutritional needs and how his development influences his behavior with food.

Countless parents of growing toddlers were always especially relieved to learn that certain behaviors surrounding toddler feeding (pushing food away, spitting food out, refusing to eat something with gusto) were actually normal, and ultimately just part of the process in becoming an independent and capable eater.

Just like so many parents I have met with over the years, you too will feel the "Ah-ha" moment when you learn how much food a toddler really needs in a day to grow and thrive, while developing a concrete understanding of what nutrients matter most and why. In addition, you will discover day-to-day prevention and management strategies for common toddler digestive issues such as diarrhea, constipation, and reflux.

Most importantly, *Give Peas a Chance* will help you

keep your sanity. I often wonder if the Shirelles were singing, "Mamma said there'll be days like this" after a long day of trying to feed a toddler. Not only will *Give Peas a Chance* provide tips for surviving this challenging time period, but it will also give parents permission to relax a little—and even enjoy being at the table next to their toddlers.

CHAPTER ONE

The "Picky" Eater

It's 7:30 a.m. The toaster waffles pop up. You lightly pat on the health-food spread and try to make the waffles kid-friendly with grapes for eyes and an engaging maple syrup smile. It's breakfast time.

You feign confidence as you walk into the living room where your two-year-old is glued to her favorite cartoon and announce, "Time to eat!" No response. Maybe she didn't hear me, you think to yourself, so you pause the TV and repeat, "Time to eat!" with the hope that she will come skipping to the table, climb into her booster seat, and gleefully yelp, "Yummy! Breakfast time!" You will then see her face shine with happiness and great satisfaction as she looks down at her plate to see the waffles smiling back at her. However, this morning, she's not buying it. You resign yourself (once again) to trying to get her to eat in whatever way possible.

Between each squeal and chant ("We did it! We did it!"), you gracefully slip in bite after bite of that smiley-face waffle, as your toddler sits propped up on the couch mindlessly eating her food without blinking an eye. This dance continues as she leaves the TV and toddles from room to room and you follow her around with her breakfast. Your mother instinct tells you *this cannot be right*, but you continue to persevere beyond all sense in the name of nutrition. Eventually, exhausted, you toss the dish with a half-eaten waffle remaining into the sink and wonder to yourself, Did she eat enough? You decide to leave some crackers out on the coffee table in case she is still hungry.

Does this sound like breakfast at your house? Does it seem that every meal is a battle to get your toddler to eat and even when she does eat, it is only from a very select list of foods? If so, you certainly seem to have a picky eater.

But, is she truly a picky eater, or simply behaving like a typical toddler?

You may be surprised to learn that her behaviors surrounding feeding *are* perfectly appropriate for her developmental stage. Once you understand why your toddler has a natural desire to eat small amounts of food on the go, rarely leaving half a butt cheek on the chair, you will feel a sense of clarity about your toddler's frustrating eating habits.

With the tools in this book, you can help your toddler learn to enjoy healthy foods that will help her to develop and grow by applying important strategies to offering scheduled meals and snacks—the essential component to raising a happy and well-nourished toddler.

TEN THINGS YOU NEED TO KNOW NOW ABOUT YOUR TODDLER'S GROWTH AND DEVELOPMENT

1. In the course of birth to the one-year mark, your infant turns into a toddler in the most rapid period of growth in a human's lifetime. Your baby (if she was born full term at thirty-eight to forty-two weeks) will essentially triple her birth weight in the first year. From birth to a year, she will have gained anywhere from twelve to seventeen pounds!

    Look at your toddler now, and try to imagine how much food she would need to eat to *triple* her current weight in the next year. Hard to imagine? Good, because she is not supposed to do that.

    On average, your toddler from age one to two will gain about four to five pounds in the year, and from age two to three will gain about four to six pounds.

2. Toddlers, particularly two- and three-year-olds, need to be given the chance to build their autonomy. You should encourage your child to feed himself, regardless of the mess it may make. Toddlers are hardwired to explore what is in front of them, and some parents find this upsetting when it comes to food. When a toddler digs his little fingers into that mound of turkey

and gravy, he genuinely thinks it is fun. More importantly, he is learning something, since this engaging activity is a key part of a toddler's development.

3. The appetite of a toddler is distinctively different from an infant's appetite: An infant's job is to eat, sleep, and drink. Nice life, right? (Kind of reminds me a little bit of college!) But after focusing so much attention on a feeding schedule during infancy, or even feeding on demand, parents might not realize that their toddler is exhibiting an appropriate appetite for her age when she takes a few bites of food and declares "all done!" There is a biological reason for a decrease in food intake between the ages of one to three, and that is a slower rate of growth. Appetite mimics rate of growth; therefore, appetite slows down. An infant's job is to eat, and a toddler's job is to eat a bit less and explore more.

4. Infants are born with an amazing ability to regulate their own food intake. This built-in sense of satiety will continue into toddlerhood, as long as you support it. Parents, determined to impose their own feeding agendas or frantic that their children are not getting "enough," often systematically undermine their child's own sense of satiety. So the next time your toddler takes a few spoonfuls of food

and declares that he is done, let it go and see what happens at the next meal. This should especially be done for toddlers who are growing normally, or along their own curve.

5. You should place more emphasis on considering the value of what your toddler eats over the course of a week, rather than from meal to meal. You can even pick a few days in a row if a week seems just too long. Remembering that her decrease in appetite is developmentally appropriate should give you some reassurance for those days that her eating doesn't seem to add up to nutrition perfection. In a day, it can be normal for a toddler to eat only one good meal out of the three. A quick example of a "good meal" would be a quarter to a half slice of whole wheat toast with butter, one slice of cheese, a handful of blueberries, plus a half cup of whole milk or a small piece of cheese.

6. At the same time that a toddler's appetite naturally decreases, his push for independence increases. This can lead to refusing to eat what you offer him, just because he has discovered the ability to say no, or because he wants to focus on what he is doing now: playing and exploring. Finding out you can be upright and mobile or crashing towers of blocks is

much more entertaining than being contained by a fastened seat or high chair.

7. Toddlers learn to identify hunger cues the way they learn to recognize the urge to use the potty (we all know how difficult this can be!). For adults, it goes something like this: stomach growls, glance up at the clock, realize it's lunchtime, find food before becoming irrational. By the time a toddler's stomach is *actually grumbling*, her blood sugar has dropped to the point of *her* becoming irrational. Trying to get an overtired, very hungry toddler to eat is what I like to refer to as the pain train. It's a lose-lose situation for everyone.

8. Toddlers know if you are overly concerned about how much they eat—and it backfires, 100 percent of the time. Developmentally, they can't help but want to test their limits with control. A typical toddler will eat *less* in those moments you want so desperately for him to eat more.

9. In the past thirty years, portions of food sold in grocery stores and restaurants have doubled, maybe even tripled, leaving even grown adults wondering what a "serving" of food actually is. Portion distortion, when a serving size of any given food, meal, or beverage

exceeds the nutritional needs of the person eating the meal, begins in the toddler stage. The amount of food a toddler is *offered* is key to a successful mealtime. So often, parents feel like their toddler is eating nothing because they have piled on grown-up portion sizes, or even quantities of food that an older sibling would eat. Start small, knowing you can always offer more if she asks for it.

HEY, MOM, LOOK AT ME!

Isn't it amazing to watch your toddler learn to do so many new things? From walking, running, jumping, hopping, skipping, climbing, and sliding—it's no wonder they have such little interest in eating.

10. Feel the love: I have come to learn that physical growth is a byproduct of many different factors well-known to scientists: nutrition, hydration, and exercise. However, after spending years of working in a neonatal intensive care unit, one of the most important contributors I've noticed is love and nurturing from a parent. So the next time your toddler throws a temper tantrum when it is time to eat, remember that is when he needs you the most.

PORTION DISTORTION

Have you ever dined at The Cheesecake Factory and ordered dessert? Or what about the number of times you hit the drive-thru of Dunkin' Donuts with your little one in tow and grabbed a muffin (essentially a small cake without frosting), a large coffee (twenty ounces of jet fuel, please), and a "juice" (twenty ounces of high-fructose corn syrup). Bags of chips, cookies, and snack crackers are bigger than ever—or should I say were bigger than ever as food companies have back-pedaled on the value bag and put efforts into making everything one hundred calories—nothing speaks more to the mishap of excessive portions than the one-hundred-calorie pack.

WARNING SIGNS OF A MORE SERIOUS PROBLEM

While many parents lament, "My child eats *nothing*," there are children for whom not eating is a true problem. As a pediatric nutritionist, when parents tell me that their toddler essentially eats nothing, I take note because there are kids who really don't eat very much at all. They seem to subsist on air, with a few bites of food throughout the day. A child who eats this way is typically not gaining weight as would be expected, and can have overall poor linear growth. Failure to gain weight or height is caused by an overall lack of adequate nutrition, which can result from one of the following circumstances:

1. The child is not receiving adequate nutrition due to limited access to food, parental neglect, or a dysfunctional parent-child relationship.

2. The child has a chronic disease that causes either improper digestion or absorption of nutrients, or a chronic disease that causes an increase in his caloric requirements beyond the child's capability to consume that increased need.

Children who fall into either of the above categories are diagnosed, often by age three, with failure to thrive (or growth failure), which can lead to serious consequences if the child is not nourished properly under supervision of a doctor and registered dietitian (RD).

There is a distinct difference between a child who has failure to thrive, and the child who has been labeled as a picky eater. So what exactly are the differences? We know that the true picky eaters stick with the same few foods time and time again and rarely (if ever) venture out to taste a new food. Or they seem to eat very small quantities of food at each meal, and usually not what you would prefer they eat. While these toddlers may gain weight at a slower rate than expected, they continue to grow appropriately. However, the picky toddler who is not "growing along his own curve" raises a red flag to you that further intervention is needed.

WHAT DOES "GROWING ALONG THE CURVE" MEAN?

Every child will grow at a different rate, and his or her growth chart will show you either a picture of progress or cause for concern. When your child visits the pediatrician, his height and weight are taken, and those values are plotted on your child's growth curve. If your child's weight and height continue to plot along the same percentile at each age, then that means he is "tracking" or growing along his own curve. For example, if your child's weight plots along the 10th percentile for his age group, then that means that 90 percent of kids the same age as your child weigh more than him, and 10 percent weigh less. This may sound like bad news, but it may not be if that is where his weight has always tracked. You need to be concerned if your child's weight decreases two or more major percentiles from a previously established growth channel. For example, if your child's weight for his age has always plotted at the 50th percentile, and now has fallen to the 10th percentile, then talk with your pediatrician and ask for a referral to a registered dietitian who specializes in pediatric nutrition (www.eatright.org; you can search for a dietitian by state and zip codes).

If you feel your child's overall growth has been less than ideal and your pediatrician has expressed concern, then your child might need to be referred to a specialist for further evaluation. In the meantime, use this book to see if you are doing everything you can to support your toddler's growth and development through nutrition, as well as doing everything you can to raise a happy and confident eater.

GETTING STARTED

Now that we have explored unique facts about growth and development of the toddler and helped to identify when special help might be needed, it is time to take stock and focus on your toddler. In order to get the most out of this book, it is essential we assess two critical factors (and set some simple and effective ground rules) that have as much of an impact on successful mealtimes as what your toddler is eating: where she sits to eat, and what her mealtime schedule looks like.

ASSESS: Where is your toddler eating?

When I sit with parents and talk about what their toddler is eating, many look surprised when I start asking about where he sits, what he sits in, and who sits with him. I admit that at first it sounds a bit like an invasion into their private home life—I am a nutritionist after all, and my questions should be about food, right? Well, actual food intake is only part of the equation in feeding success. I can't help families unless I know this information, as it impacts the toddler's ability to eat well. Simply stated, where your child eats is as important as what he eats. Ask yourself the following questions:

- Is he able to see and reach what he is eating?
- Is he sitting at a table in a chair that secures him and supports his ability to feed himself? Or are you following him around the house with bites of food for most meals?
- Are you, the parent, sitting, eating, and interacting with your child while assisting with feeding?
- Does your family sit at a dining or kitchen table that fosters a sense of mealtime?
- Are distractions such as phones, television, emails, etc., minimized during mealtimes?

If you answered yes to all of these questions, then you are off to a good start in regard to where your toddler should be eating. However, if you answered no to even one of the questions, then more work needs to be done with your eating routine. Follow the guidelines below to best support your toddler:

- Your child should sit at a table in a chair that secures her and supports her ability to self-feed. This allows her to feel well balanced and included as part of the family table.

- Rather than facing an exasperated adult trying to shove a spoon in her mouth, your child should be able to face family members while eating. Both trust and autonomy are involved here. If she is secure while she is eating, she will be able to develop independent feeding skills, and trust continues to develop as she watches others eat and feed themselves.

- No toddler can be expected to sit for any meal for more than ten minutes. If you are one of the lucky parents who has a toddler who enjoys sitting at the table with others for longer, by no means do you have to end her table time once ten minutes passes. However, if you find you are struggling to keep your toddler at the table, then allowing ten minutes of table time is completely acceptable and plenty of time for your toddler to eat enough of her meal and be nourished.

- I have met many families with multiple children who tell me it is house rules to wait until everyone is finished before hopping down from the table. This is not an unreasonable expectation for an older toddler, but could be a challenge for a younger one.

- If you make a toddler sit for longer than he can, he might not want to come back. If you find he can't sit for five minutes, then you have to focus your attention on setting realistic expectations and working on them at every meal. I have found it useful to ignore the "I'm done" remark and simply start a new conversation or ask a silly question that might engage the toddler. This is especially helpful at dinnertime since it is the hardest meal to get through—the day has been long and everyone is tired.

- The parent should be sitting, eating, and interacting with the toddler while assisting with feeding when needed. If you are not eating too, then you are spending too much effort trying to feed your toddler. The family table is a place toddlers need to learn to come to with pleasure. Studies abound about the positive effects of eating together as a family—and it is never too early (or late!) to start.

ASSESS: What is your feeding routine or schedule?

We all know toddlers thrive on structure and routine and look to adults to set limits to make them feel "safe," but many parents have confessed they just don't feel their toddler can independently eat enough for the day if limits are set by maintaining a feeding schedule. From the parents' perspective, this makes sense: how can you say no to a toddler asking for food *to eat*, when most of the time you are trying so hard to *get him to eat*? Saying no to toddlers begging for food in between meals is not easy. However, if you find you are handing out food to your toddler every one to two hours each day, then he won't reap the benefits of the most powerful weapon against picky eating: physical hunger.

GOT HUNGER?

As a species, we are meant to get hungry. It is a biological intention that our bodies rely on ultimately for survival. The feeling of an empty stomach or perhaps stomach growling are identifiable signs of hunger; even our mood can change when we feel hungry. In addition to the physical signs of hunger, there is a strong cognitive component that mostly results from learned behaviors. For example, your toddler will know it's lunchtime if you eat at right about the same time every day, simply because her body has been trained to do so.

It seems that parents today are afraid to allow their child to get hungry. Snacks are carried everywhere, and unfortunately, snacks can be *bought* everywhere. Honestly, it's insane. I am not saying snacks are bad—in fact, planned snacks are good and necessary for ages one to three. But research has shown that kids who graze all day may take in up to 50 percent fewer calories in a day than if on a schedule. Grazing also deprives the toddler of motivation to try new foods.

If you feel that you are using snacks to quell a tired or frustrated toddler more often than not, then you need to reexamine your feeding schedule and be sure to say no when you know your child is not hungry and simply being a toddler.

Parents and grandparents have told me numerous times that having *planned* snacks that are small in portion and healthy (think: fruits, a cheese stick, peanut butter crackers, four ounces of milk with two graham crackers, cereal and milk) have helped their toddlers gain weight steadily without squelching their appetite for a main meal.

A typical feeding schedule for a toddler should look like this:

Breakfast: 7:00–7:30 a.m.
Snack: 9:30–10:00 a.m.
Lunch: 11:30 a.m.–12:30 p.m.
Afternoon nap
Snack: 2:30–3:30 p.m.
Dinner: 5:00–6:00 p.m.
Bedtime snack: 7:00–7:30 p.m.
Brush teeth, story, bed

A regular schedule promotes a healthy relationship with food, and gives the toddler the opportunity to eat the amount of food she wants, knowing that the next meal (or snack) is not too far away. Many parents find reminding their toddler that he can't eat again until snack time is helpful. Try using positive phrases like, "Are you sure you are done? We can't eat again until snack time. You might get hungry before then and have to wait." If he chooses not to eat more than two bites of Cheerios, then breakfast is over. For example, if your toddler comes to eat breakfast and takes two bites of food and then thirty minutes later wants a snack, you might remind him not to rush through his breakfast the next time.

Most importantly, stay tuned in to your toddler's hunger rhythm and support her natural hunger cues. Day after day, if you find that your three-year-old just can't stomach a big breakfast at seven o'clock in the morning, then offer something small (e.g., half a slice of whole wheat toast with cream cheese or a cereal bar) and know she will most likely be hungry again between nine and nine-thirty. Allowing some flexibility surrounding feeding schedules will help your toddler trust you and help her to develop autonomy with eating.

A word about activity and hunger: premeal exercise. It makes a world of difference for kids of all ages to be outside playing before mealtime rather than to be plopped in front of the computer or in front of the TV. Kids are much more interested in coming and sitting down at the table if they have not been sitting for the past hour doing nothing. Even for older toddlers, staying active doing an art project will keep their focus on something other than begging for snacks before dinner.

Josh's Story

This is a great example from a family I spent a lot of time with helping them make small changes to their very hectic weekend schedule.

Joshua was a very active three-year-old boy whose parents themselves had a limited diet—certain foods they avoided altogether for health reasons, and others they just simply did not eat. Both parents worked outside the home and relied on Josh's day-care provider to feed two of the three meals to him as well as snacks. He had been gaining weight at a slow pace and his doctor expressed concern that his weight gain was "less than ideal," and referred them to our clinic.

His parents were upset because they felt helpless since he ate most meals at his day-care center five days a week. On weekends, their schedules were packed with activities for all three of their children, so nobody really paid attention to what anybody was eating. When I asked them to describe a typical day of eating for Joshua, it went something like this:

7:00 a.m. Wake up.

7:30 a.m. Offered plain waffle—he refused.

8:00 a.m. Joshua asks for **waffle** now that he is "hungry" and walks around eating it until two-thirds of it is gone.

8:45 a.m. Family packs up for a soccer game; Joshua brings **pretzels** with him and devours the whole bag in the car.

9:30 a.m. At the soccer game, he meets some friends and they have brought **donut holes**, and he eats about four.

11:30 a.m. At home, lunch is made, but he does not eat much because he is "not hungry."

1:00 p.m. Asks for lunch now; parents oblige and begin to make him macaroni and cheese, but he is so hungry that he can't wait for the mac and cheese, so he eats **crackers** while he is waiting. Once the macaroni and cheese is cooked and on the plate, he sits for two minutes, takes three bites (not too bad), and off he goes.

1:45 p.m. Complains of hunger, offered **fruit snacks**, accepts.

3:00 p.m. Eats a few bites of a **bagel** with peanut butter that Mom is snacking on.

4:00 p.m. Asks for milk because he is thirsty—drinks one cup.

5:30 p.m. Dinnertime; he does well and eats some chicken and potato with a few bites of peas.

7:00 p.m. Wants a snack and eats **Teddy Grahams**.

If you closely take a look at this pattern of eating you will see that what Josh is eating most of (in bold) are snack-type foods, with very little calcium, vitamin A, protein, and fat. This regular lack of nutrients in Josh's eating pattern contributed to the slow weight gain his doctor highlighted. Let's take a look at how Josh's nutritional status can be improved:

BEFORE	AFTER
7:30 A.M. Offered plain waffle—he refused. **8:00 A.M.** Joshua asks for waffle now that he is "hungry" and walks around eating it until two-thirds of it is gone.	**8:00 A.M.** Serve waffle with some butter and a favorite fruit. Pour half a cup of milk for him to drink and pour yourself a cup of coffee and sit down with him. Better yet, eat breakfast yourself.
8:45 A.M. Family packs up for a soccer game; Joshua brings pretzels with him and devours the whole bag in the car.	**8:45 A.M.** Ask Josh what he would like to bring for a snack, and ask him if he wants to pack it in a special sack. Remind him that he will be happy to have the snack at soccer because he will be hungry from running around. Put special bag in the car and allow Josh to carry his water bottle.

BEFORE	AFTER
9:30 A.M. At the soccer game, he meets some friends and they have brought donut holes, which he eats about four of.	**9:30 A.M.:** Remind Josh that he brought his own snack so he should only take two donut holes today. Josh forgets about his snack, which is fine.
1:45 P.M. Complains of hunger, offered fruit snacks, accepts.	**12:30 P.M.** Offer fruit snacks for dessert after proper food.
3:00 P.M. Eats a few bites of a bagel with peanut butter that Mom is snacking on. **4.00 P.M.** Asks for milk because he is thirsty— drinks one cup.	**3:00 P.M.** Announce that it is snack time and serve half a bagel with peanut butter. Offer milk.
5:30 P.M. He does well at dinnertime and eats some chicken and potato with a few bites of peas.	**5:30 P.M.** Continue dinner routine. Make attempts to direct talk to keep Josh at the table. Add a safety food or whole wheat bread and butter.
7:00 P.M. Asks for Teddy Grahams for a snack.	**7:00 P.M.** Serve pudding with Teddy Grahams for a snack.

By implementing the changes you see in the "After" column, Josh's parents would be keeping a better schedule that supports his hunger and also minimizes the amount of empty-calorie, snack-type food. Dairy has been added with meals, as well as fruits and vegetables. Repeatedly exposing Josh to this kind of weekend routine will help the parents set simple boundaries for Josh that will in turn make him feel better and keep his body weight on track. This type of plan will also empower the parents to give some guidance for the day-care provider in regards to regulation of meals and snacks.

Now that we have assessed the how, when, and where of your toddler's eating, it's time to look at exactly *what* she is eating. Specifically, let's look at what kinds of foods she chooses and how much she actually eats.

WHAT *IS* YOUR TODDLER EATING?

Many parents find a mismatch between the food their toddler is eating and what they think he should be consuming at every meal. The confusion lies with both the amount of food eaten as well as the variety of foods selected. Because every toddler is different, with varying caloric needs, there is no one-size-fits-all in terms of the quantities of food that your child should be consuming. It would be a disservice for me to simply tell you specific quantities that would serve for every toddler.

While I can give you guidelines about quantities and information on nutritious foods, it is more important for you to take stock and assess your current situation to determine what will work best for you and your toddler. In the following pages you will be asked to:

- take a close look at what he is eating
- identify textures and types of food he gravitates to (or most readily accepts)

I will then:

- provide insight on how to introduce new foods
- provide tools to help your toddler expand the variety in his diet

The food list: taking stock

In order to get a true sense of what your child is eating, take five or ten minutes to write down everything that she is willing to eat. This includes table food, snacks, drinks, desserts, candies, spices, condiments, vitamins—everything. Even if she has tried the particular food only once or twice, write it down.

This activity will:

- give you reassurance that your toddler has an average (or better yet) above average variety in her diet

- help you identify possible trends in what your toddler will eat
- give you ideas for new foods to introduce to your toddler

Don't categorize the foods or put them in groups; simply write down everything in a list as it comes to you.

DEFINING VARIETY

If your toddler has fifteen foods in his diet that he willingly eats, then he has a decent variety of choices. Toddlers who like four to five foods from each of the food groups are the most likely to have a balanced diet.

This means food from the fruit/vegetable group, grains, dairy, and proteins (meats).

If at least half of the foods your toddler enjoys are snack-type foods, then there is work to be done!

Be sure to include beverages as well as fats that would be added to foods or used in cooking (for example, oils, butter, margarines, spreads). Next, I want you to look at your list and see if you can expand it. Go back through the list and in the second column add specific varieties of each food your child eats. For example, if you wrote "bread," make separate entries for each type or variety of bread your child currently eats. Be sure to note as well if your child prefers a specific form of any given food (for example, cooked carrots versus raw, breaded chicken versus skinless).

FOODS	SPECIFIC FOODS

See the examples below for guidance:

FOODS	SPECIFIC FOODS
Bread	Wheat bread, bakery Italian bread, toasted English muffin
Apples	Granny Smith, Fuji, dried apples
Cereal	Cheerios, Rice Chex, Kix
Cheese	American, cheddar, cream cheese
Turkey	Roasted, deli
Pasta	Ziti, rotini
Butter	Unsalted, Smart Balance

What this exercise does is shift your perception about your toddler and food. When you look at the left-hand column, it is easy to say there is not much there. But if you count the number of foods in the right-hand column, you can see that the list has expanded from seven foods to eighteen without adding anything new. This new perspective allows you to see foods differently and can take some pressure off in the quest for nutrition perfection. You might be saying, "Turkey is turkey, no matter how you slice it," but it's not. Food comes in so many forms and textures and can be prepared in so many different ways that you must allow yourself to recognize even the slightest differences in foods that might appear to be the same in order to successfully expand your child's diet.

The food list: identify trends

- Does he like crunchy, salty foods, or does he prefer sweet and soft?
- Is he a meat-eater, or does he choose dairy-based foods over meats?
- Does he like to drink liquid more than eat solids?
- Does he select hot (oatmeal, pizza) more often than cold (Cheerios, ham and cheese)?
- Does he typically choose fruits over vegetables?
- Does he like snack foods or proper food?

"PROPER" FOOD DEFINED

A wonderful European mother I knew often told her kids when they were asking for snacks that they needed "proper food" first. I loved the phrase immediately. What a fantastic yet simple way to gently remind your toddler that certain foods are better than others without using the phrase "that is bad for you." Proper food encompasses foods that are nutrient-dense and filling. That means they have some protein, carbohydrate, and fat. Here are some good examples:

Meats with vegetables

Pasta with beans and olive oil

Hummus or cheese with crackers

Yogurt and fruit

Macaroni and cheese

Pizza (by the slice, bagel, English muffin)

Cereal and milk

Deli turkey roll-ups and semi-strained
  vegetable soup

Spaghetti and meatballs

Cheese ravioli

Omelet with cheese

Flour tortilla with melted cheese and thinly
  spread refried beans

Your list may reflect that your toddler always accepts fruits willingly, but will only eat cooked carrots for vegetables. Or maybe you can see that your toddler refuses meat unless it is breaded, such as in the form of a chicken nugget. Or maybe it is obvious that your toddler loves to drink milk and water, but does not eat much solid food other than snacks like Goldfish or pretzels. Whatever trend you may have identified, this will become the starting point for expanding your child's diet. It is extremely important to understand that, on average, it can take a toddler nine to fifteen times to be exposed to one food before she is willing to accept it on a regular basis. Notice I used the word *exposed*. Your toddler may or may not eat the food nine times; she simply has to be offered it.

There is no doubt that simply exposing a toddler to food is the most frustrating piece of advice for parents to swallow; you have taken time to plan, shop, and prepare a meal, and by God, you want your tot to eat it. I myself plead guilty to attempting to coerce a toddler to try a new food by bribing with a favorite dessert. It happens. The trick is to resist the impulse to "get him to eat" and embrace the concept of exposing him to new foods as often as a few times per week. Find comfort with the idea that modeling good eating habits yourself, e.g., "I am eating my vegetables, you eat yours," goes a long way toward food acceptance.

Remain neutral while eating and try to enjoy your meal while he takes a few bites of whatever is on his plate. I know, this is much easier said than done, but consider the concept of what I like to call "the safety food": a safety food is one food that you are certain your toddler will accept—something familiar and likeable. When your toddler comes to the table and finds new food on his plate, the safety food serves to disarm that immediate protest or reaction of panic that is often responsible for the cascade of dinnertime battles that are customary to so many when presenting something untried. Your toddler might have fewer objections once his eye catches the safety food. Ideally, he might settle into his seat with the reassurance that there is something on the table he likes, and the option to try the new food.

Brooke's Story

Brooke was a thirteen-month-old who suffered from reflux as an infant, which consequently led her to have some food aversions and difficulty gaining weight. She was recently started on medication to help minimize the discomfort associated with reflux. These medications are not meant to stop the regurgitation (or vomiting) from happening; they work to protect the esophagus (the tube that connects your mouth to your stomach) from irritating, acidic stomach contents. Brooke's mom was very anxious about her lack of weight gain and became so focused on the calorically dense foods that we had recommended when she was six months old that she never felt comfortable trying anything new. She stuck to a rigid list of what Brooke could "have" to help her gain weight, and that was it. Brooke was receiving a very balanced diet; however, she became so bored with what she was offered that she stopped eating. When I asked Brooke's mom what her daughter's typical lunch was, she told me Brooke ate a full-fat yogurt (made with whole milk), the same flavor every day. She never tried giving Brooke a new flavor because she had always accepted this one—and her mom, of course, wanted Brooke to eat something nutritionally dense and loaded with calcium. I asked her to buy one new flavor and offer that instead of the usual, and to vary Brooke's lunch by adding some whole-grain crackers with spreadable cheese and fruit.

After about three attempts with trying new flavors of yogurt, Brooke accepted one new flavored yogurt, in addition to the whole-grain crackers and spreadable cheese—and after about three weeks, went back to eating the original flavor as well. The yogurt became part of a meal—not an obligatory load of bone-building calcium. Brooke was happier because she was introduced to new foods that she quite enjoyed, and she was still maintaining her weight—which made her mom happy.

The food list expanded

To help you find new foods your toddler will like based on similarities to foods he already eats, use the chart below as a starting place for diet expansion. Refer to the food list you made for your child. It should help guide you with selecting textures and tastes your toddler gravitates to.

CRUNCHY/ SALTY	SWEET/ SQUISHY	SOFT MEATS/ PROTEINS
Chips: Terra Stix, Baked Cheetos, Pirate's Booty, Veggie Stix, Pretzel Stix, Pop Chips	Sweet breads: banana, zucchini, pumpkin	Small meatballs cooked in sauce
Dried cereal: Rice Chex, Honey Kix, Cheerios (Multigrain, Original), Life	Muffins: berry, banana, corn, lemon poppyseed	Strained meat-based soups
Letter cookies	Pancakes, crepes	Strained pot pies
Multigrain crackers	French toast	Diced breakfast sausages
Mini rice cakes	Cereal bars, broken in small pieces	Beef ravioli

CRUNCHY/ SALTY	SWEET/ SQUISHY	SOFT MEATS/ PROTEINS
Garlic bread	Waffles with butter	Fish sticks
Tater Tots	Frozen pizza cooked soft, cut in cubes	Hot dogs cut in small pieces without skin
Breaded chicken, pork, or fish	Freeze-dried fruits	Salmon cakes

DAIRY	FULL OF FLAVOR	FOODS THAT MUSH IN THE MOUTH
Yogurt	Hummus	Well-cooked macaroni and cheese or well-cooked small pastas
Cottage cheese	Boxed stuffing mix cooked as directed—rolled into balls	Buttered grilled cheese, cut in cubes
Cream cheese	Falafel	French fries (oven-baked)
Cheese spreads	Pasta Alfredo	Oven-baked chicken nuggets, cut in cubes

DAIRY	FULL OF FLAVOR	FOODS THAT MUSH IN THE MOUTH
Ricotta cheese	Baby quiche	Eggplant Parmesan
Yogurt smoothie	Refried beans	Noodle pudding (kugel)
Shredded, sliced, or cubed cheeses	Guacamole	Potato pancakes, pierogies
Pudding	Beef stew, strained	Lasagna or stuffed shells

HOW TO USE THIS CHART: If your toddler prefers pancakes for breakfast, then you can choose a food from the chart above in the same column as pancakes—in this case you would look under the column "sweet and squishy." Or if your list reflects that your child is drinking a lot of milk throughout the day and squeezing by on snack foods, then you want to try and offer a different dairy-based food, such as pudding or a yogurt smoothie. The goal is to try and identify foods that are similar in texture and consistency to foods that he already accepts and that have the same "mouth feel." It is also important to think about what flavors your child gravitates to; if he seems to really like banana bread, then you need to key in on that and try Banana Nut

Cheerios in place of plain Cheerios, banana-flavored pudding, banana cream pie, or even banana pancakes. The familiar and accepted flavor of banana may be a bridge to a new texture or food acceptance.

INTRODUCING NEW FOODS

Now that we have talked about how to approach expanding your toddler's food choices, we need to talk about introducing new foods. This may seem like a simple task—put plate in front of toddler and say "dinnertime." But for many of you readers, things probably have not gone so smoothly. I don't need to tell you that toddlers can be very set in their ways about what foods they are willing to eat. New foods are often met with a flat-out refusal to eat or even taste it.

The trick is to offer it without forcing it on her. Here's how:

- Put the food in front of her in small, manageable pieces that will be easy for her to eat without choking.
- Offer the food in small quantities so she does not get discouraged or overwhelmed.
- Offer the food with a safety food and as part of a meal, as discussed earlier in this chapter. Remember that a safety food is one food that you are certain your toddler will accept—something familiar and likeable. For example, if you are trying to expose your toddler

to meat, pair it with her favorite fruit or vegetable and a starch (e.g., watermelon and French fries).

- Allow your toddler to touch and play with that food, even if it means putting it in her mouth and then spitting it out.
- Serve the same food to all at the table, so your toddler will see other people eating what she is being served.
- Keep conversation pleasant and resist the urge to coax her to eat.

If after two minutes your toddler says the dreaded "I'm done," ignore her and attempt to engage her to talk about something she did that day. Do not attempt to overzealously keep her at the table or set "rules" for what else she has to eat before she gets down. Remember to use ten minutes as a goal to work up to, which will often happen in increasing increments of about two to three minutes. For example, if your toddler only seems to sit for about five minutes, then work toward seven, then ten.

CONSEQUENCES OF "FORCING" FOOD

Many parents come to my office with their own personal history of food battles. Often I learn that one parent, as a child, might have been made to "clean his plate" with each and every meal. Despite knowing how awful this made them feel when they were little, the strategy is simply what they "know" to do as parents now. Forcing food into a toddler's mouth can vary from a benign attempt to get calories into him (e.g., coaxing a spoon or bottle into her mouth), or can be an extreme form of punishment (e.g., not allowing your toddler to leave the table until his plate is cleaned or punishing him for not eating).

In either circumstance, I urge you to resist the temptation to "make" or "force" your toddler to eat. Forcing food has an extensive list of long-term consequences associated with it, the most important one being interfering with the ability to decide for yourself when you are full. This disruption can lead to binge eating and hoarding food (think obesity), or for some kids, a genuine fear of eating.

In short, forcing food can cause long-term emotional baggage for both the child and the parent.

So many parents of "smaller" toddlers will tell me they often try and distract their toddler to "finish" his plate or bowl of food. If you find you are distracting your toddler and spooning food into his mouth beyond when he has tried to throw down the red flag, take a look below at ways your toddler will tell you he is full:

1. Turns head away from spoon.
2. Purses or closes lips when food comes to mouth.
3. Pushes bowl or spoon away with hand.
4. Shakes head no.
5. Verbalizes "No more!" or "All done."

Jenny's Story

Three-year-old Jenny was a picky eater who often refused "proper food" in the name of cheese puffs. Her mother was very upset about this as she considered them to be a "junk food." When I asked Mom how Jenny was introduced to them, she told me her mother-in-law often gave them to Jenny. Jenny would then whine for cheese puffs every evening before dinner, like clockwork. After Mom repeatedly said "no" and dealt with the resulting temper tantrum, when it was actually time to sit down for dinner, both Mom and Jenny were exhausted. Even worse, Jenny would refuse to eat because she had her heart set on those cheese puffs.

I asked Mom if she ever broke down and gave them to Jenny before dinner, and she said yes. Then I asked Mom if she ever put some on Jenny's plate *at* dinner—and she looked at me in horror. I explained that if she added a few cheese puffs to her plate as the carbohydrate source next to some baked chicken and a favored fruit and vegetable, Jenny might not see them as being so special, and willingly come to dinner. In fact, she might also take a few bites of the main meal in the meantime. After a few weeks of getting cheese puffs with dinner, Jenny didn't ask for them as much because she knew she could have them. Eventually, Mom was able to swap out the cheese puffs at dinner with mashed potatoes or small cooked pasta shells and offer the cheese puffs as one of the choices for an after-dinner snack.

Now that we have set the ground rules surrounding toddler feeding and have a handle on what your toddler eats now, the next chapter will expand on food exposure and introducing foods with special attention to the transition from pureed jar foods to proper table food.

CHAPTER TWO

Moving Beyond the Jar

Introducing Your Tater Tot to Table Foods

If you are the parent of a toddler, jarred foods might already be a thing of the past. However, many families I see in my practice struggle with letting go of jarred foods (particularly for the twelve- to twenty-month-old) and find themselves moving into prepackaged toddler meals, or even hanging on to stage three jars of thick purees. As I listened to these parents, it became evident that they were afraid to let go of the jars and move to table food, because they just didn't feel their toddlers could eat enough on their own.

This parental overcompensation often resulted in

1. **Limited diet expansion**: Parents become reluctant to attempt expanding their toddler's diet to include more table food. Many often told me they felt their toddler just wouldn't eat well if they offered anything other than jars. This undermined the parents' perception of their own ability to cook "real food" for their toddler.

2. **Limited opportunities**: Practice makes perfect, right? A toddler needs multiple opportunities through the

first three years of his life to practice eating table foods. Given enough practice, he will advance faster to a more complex diet, and move into eating what the whole family eats (e.g., proper food).

3. **Interfering with self-regulation of appetite**: Toddlers have the right to learn how much table food makes them feel full and should not be forced to choke down half of a jar of stage three chicken and stars because it makes us (the parent) feel better. As we are all very aware of the increasing prevalence of pediatric obesity, we must covet one of the human body's greatest defenses against obesity: the ability to feel full.

While you are considering the above information, read below as to how the food industry is making it harder for you to move away from jarred or toddler foods.

THE INDUSTRY

Baby-food companies are continually seeking ways to maintain or expand their sales base. Gerber and Beech-Nut have extended their product lines to include foods for toddlers—enticing one of the most desperate groups of parents on the planet. Just as your infant is turning ten months old, trying to declare her independence, and learning to feed herself (insert image of baby dumping out mush onto the floor and screeching), mothers across the country are opening their mailboxes to direct mail promotions for prepackaged foods for toddlers ages one to three years. Companies such as Gerber, Heinz, and Beech-Nut market the concept that prepared prepackaged foods provide peace of mind for parents struggling with picky eaters, leaving many to feel less motivated to simply serve what they are cooking. This can lead parents to believe that these perfectly portioned, microwavable, and shelf-stable meals are better than adult table food due to a toddler's special growing needs. Sure, the meals are calculated to include a decent amount of protein and calcium, but they lack the fat, calories, and antioxidants that fresh, homemade food would provide. Essentially, what the toddler meal does is demystify the "did he eat enough?" phenomenon for new parents: "If my toddler eats this whole container, then he is good to go." But is he? What parents may not realize is that the baby food market is a $750-million industry, *with the best potential new growth coming in the toddler food segment.*

Are toddler foods really necessary, though? Take a look at the following table, which compares prepared toddler foods with good alternatives made right in your very own kitchen:

TODDLER MEALS OR STAGE THREE JARRED FOOD	YUMMY TABLE FOOD EQUIVALENT
Sweet potatoes	Smashed sweet potatoes with butter and cinnamon
Macaroni and beef	Three-cheese meat lasagna with chopped spinach and basil
Turkey dinner	Shredded pieces of white meat turkey tossed in gravy; side of mashed potatoes and soft-cooked carrot cubes with butter
Chicken and stars	Homemade chicken noodle soup with acini de pepe (very small) noodles and peas, strained well
Beef and tomato cheese ravioli	Mama Rosa's cheese or beef ravioli with soft-cooked diced green beans and olive oil
Garden vegetables with pasta and tomato sauce	Barilla mini penne or small shells with finely chopped soft-cooked broccoli, tossed in 2 tablespoons chicken broth, and 1 tablespoon tomato sauce and butter

TODDLER MEALS OR STAGE THREE JARRED FOOD	YUMMY TABLE FOOD EQUIVALENT
Chicken and pasta wheel pick-ups	Cubed cooked chicken cutlets with a side of pasta pinwheels with parmesan and butter
Creamy chicken and noodles	Frozen chicken pot pie, with the crust removed and the inside strained a bit
Fruit melts or fruit snacks	Fresh blueberries, cut in half

When you look at this table, first ask yourself, what would you rather eat? Then consider the following:

1. Heinz and Gerber add significant amounts of water and thickening agents (flours and chemically modified starches) to more than half of their twenty-five products for babies over six months. In fact, single ingredient stage one foods for babies less than six months are nutritionally superior, as less water is added and fillers are omitted (source: Center for Science in the Public Interest/CSPI).

2. Prepared jars of food are made with predominantly fruits, vegetables, and protein, but they are limited

in calcium as well as necessary healthy fats. When you consider the foods on the right side of the chart, you see that dairy and fat can be added easily to improve nutritional quality—and flavor.

3. Stage three jarred foods are mixed textures and could be a disaster with a picky toddler who is texture sensitive, or even with one that is not. When you spoon a thick puree into a toddler's mouth, they can basically swallow it as is—very reassuring and a confidence builder, especially for the younger toddler who is still experimenting with food.

    However, if the next bite has a landmine of turkey or apple in it, the toddler may not know how to separate the texture in her mouth, and either gag or choke on the chunk until it slides down, or simply spit out the chunk and attempt to swallow the puree. Immediately she begins to lose confidence in her capability to eat and becomes frustrated. This leads to spitting out the food, and for most toddlers, almost always marks the end of mealtime altogether. If you have had similar frustrations, use the chart of table food equivalents to guide you in finding good alternatives to the stage three jar of baby food.

4. Toddler entrées can be low in total calories and fat. If your toddler is drinking sixteen ounces per day

(or two cups) of one percent milk and eating three commercially prepared entrées per day, he is only meeting about 60 percent of his calorie needs and 20 percent of his fat requirements. This leaves a toddler hungry, looking to fill in the blanks with snacks that are typically void of any nutritional value.

Gerber and Heinz make about 120 different baby foods and sell over 230 million units of baby food annually. This leaves many parents feeling less motivated to try real table food (e.g., what they actually are eating for dinner) with their tot since there is something premade that is "nutritionally complete." As you can see from the chart, there are many healthy, easy foods parents can feel good about quickly preparing for their toddler, and serve on a regular basis.

So how do commercially prepared baby foods and toddler meals measure up in quantity to proper food equivalents? Take a look at the following chart.

BABY OR TODDLER FOOD	PROPER FOOD EQUIVALENT
4-ounce jar of fruit or vegetable (stage two)	About 6 tablespoons of the real food equivalent
6-ounce jar of vegetable or fruit (stage three)	About 8 tablespoons of the real food equivalent

BABY OR TODDLER FOOD	PROPER FOOD EQUIVALENT
6-ounce jar meat and vegetable dinner (stage three)	1 tablespoon oven roasted turkey, shredded 4 tablespoons mashed yamanana (cooked yams with ¼ of a ripe banana mashed in) 1 teaspoon butter
Toddler meal (Gerber Graduate)	1 tablespoon cut up chicken 3–4 spoons of pasta noodles + ½ teaspoon olive oil or butter 2 broccoli trees with stems cut off

Despite the remarkable changes in the variety of baby and toddler foods available today, food from a family meal will always taste better and be nutritionally superior for your toddler. And remember, if you find yourself relying on toddler meals every once in a while, that is OK. Just know that the foods listed on the right will offer more flavor (think taste expansion), and food that tastes good is another secret weapon against picky eating.

One caveat though: if your twelve- to fifteen-month-old is truly struggling to gain weight and the only thing for lunch she wants to have is a big jar of Earth's Best Organic Turkey and Sweet Potatoes, then just go with it. Many parents come into my office and tell me that they offer table foods in small pieces and finish off the meal with a four- to six-ounce jar of baby food—this is fine for that age group, as not every toddler will adjust to table foods at the same pace. What I urge you to do is focus on incorporating some more semi-solid foods on her high chair tray that are very easy to "manage in the mouth" and play with to practice the skill of advancing textures. Good examples would be:

FRUITS	SOFT-COOKED VEGGIES	PROTEINS	CARBS
Blueberries cut in half	Carrot cubes Green beans cut in half	Small beans: pinto, baby red kidney, black, baked	Small pasta noodles: ditalini, piccolini by Barilla in chicken broth; Annie's pasta and stars
Dole diced peaches or apples packed in 100% fruit juice	Sweet potato, baked and cubed	Chopped hard-boiled egg	Soft-cooked French fries; Dr. Praeger's Potato Littles, Broccoli Littles, or spinach pancakes; Trader Joe's potato pancakes

FRUITS	SOFT-COOKED VEGGIES	PROTEINS	CARBS
Banana wheels	Spring peas (give them a chance please!)	Small pieces of chopped chicken, shredded chicken, beef, pork or turkey, fish	Whole wheat toast strips with butter
Soft melon cut in tiny cubes	Baby broccoli or Broccoli Littles	Small cheese cubes	Crackers, puffs, dry cereals
Soft cubed pears	Creamed spinach	Baked, extra-firm tofu	Cubed pieces of sweet breads

Remember to offer these foods frequently, at least once a day but up to every meal, as food exposure is the key to food acceptance.

Abby's Story

Three-year-old Abby had two working parents and was in day care five days a week for eight hours a day. She was referred by her pediatrician to our office for slow weight gain. Over the past year, she had gone from the 25th percentile in weight for age down to the 10th percentile. Her mom Stacy was obviously concerned and had kept a food journal of what Abby was eating for two full weeks.

Each night for dinner, Stacy had jotted down "Graduates," and wrote down three different varieties over the span of two weeks. When I asked Mom what she and her husband ate for dinner, she went on to explain that she was not the best cook, so they often ate some kind of baked chicken, a fruit, and a vegetable for dinner. When I asked why she didn't offer what she was making to Abby, she simply said it was not "nutritious" enough for her. As we talked more, I learned that Abby had been eating less and less with each toddler meal, due to what Mom said was "lack of interest." Stacy also confessed she often ended up packing them for her lunch at day care as well due to their convenience.

What Stacy didn't realize was that the calories offered in many prepackaged meals are not hefty enough for an older toddler day in and day out, unless you are adding something to the meal such as a cheese stick, milk, and/or a yogurt. Not to mention that the taste can be less than ideal compared to real food (just like many of the low-calorie frozen meals we have all bought at one point or another!).

I reassured Stacy that what she was making was better for Abby and offered her a challenge to learn to expand her cooking skills so everyone would benefit from a variety of nutritious meals. When they came back to the office for a follow-up visit, Mom had found a few reliable websites for recipes, subscribed to a monthly magazine offering recipes for the whole family, and she even took a few cooking classes at a local retail store. Abby was doing much better at mealtimes, gaining weight, and became the sous-chef of the house by completing simple tasks like tearing lettuce, sprinkling cheese, and setting the table.

MOVING TO TABLE FOOD: ALLERGIES, INTOLERANCES, AND CHOKING HAZARDS

With a dramatic increase in the number of children developing food allergies, some of which can be life-threatening, I answer multiple questions a week about what foods are safe to introduce to toddlers. I can certainly empathize with all of these parents. Food has never been so confusing. It has been estimated that four out of every one hundred children have a food allergy, with the largest number of children affected being less than five years of age. Parents ask about the whens of including foods from strawberries to citrus fruits and egg whites to honey. What many parents might not know is that eight types of food account for over 90 percent of allergic reactions. These are milk, peanuts, eggs, treenuts, fish, soy, wheat, and shellfish.

The good news is that in 2008, the American Academy of Pediatrics (AAP) released a report stating that there was not enough evidence to support delaying the introduction of complementary foods beyond four to six months of age, with hopes to prevent the development of a food allergy. In addition, current evidence does not support a major role for maternal dietary restriction during pregnancy or lactation to prevent allergy. This is true even for mothers who are pregnant and nursing. If, however, you already have a child with food allergies and are concerned about your infant developing one, talk with your pediatrician about the benefits of avoiding that particular food. You will find that many doctors feel strongly about early introduction of these foods to *avoid* developing an allergy. And remember, introducing one new food every three to five days is a good rule of thumb to follow. If your toddler does have a reaction, you will know which food is responsible. More importantly, any kind of reaction might be dose-dependent, meaning he might not react until a second or third exposure. Take a look below at the list of foods parents ask about most frequently.

Egg: Many parents receive conflicting advice about when it is safe to introduce cooked egg yolk alone versus the whole egg. It is safe to introduce cooked egg yolk alone by six or seven months of age and the white next by twelve months of age. I always think it is a good idea to offer foods that have the whole egg cooked into it around nine or ten months. This would include things like cookies, meatballs, muffins, pancakes, French toast, etc. Never give your baby or toddler raw egg or foods that contain raw egg.

Strawberries: Many parents are fearful of giving fresh strawberries to their toddler, as strawberries have been

SIGNS OF AN ALLERGIC REACTION

It is important to know what to look for as a sign that your toddler may be having an allergic reaction to a food you have introduced. Many parents often report red blotchy smears around their toddler's mouth, usually within thirty minutes of feeding. This can be a contact reaction to the food actually touching the toddler's face for a period of time—especially if you are (hopefully) allowing him to become super messy. The rash often goes away after the toddler is clean and done eating.

However, true signs of a food allergy would include the development of hives (small raised bumps), a rash that starts on the face and spreads down the trunk of the body, unusual irritability, runny nose and/or "cold-like symptoms," diarrhea, vomiting, or, worst-case scenario, difficulty breathing. It is always best to call your pediatrician to report any concerns and bring your child in to be looked at if warranted.

said to cause allergic reactions in some highly atopic/sensitive babies. Some doctors have put the kibosh on offering fresh strawberries until the baby is one year old, while some will give the green light for cooked or heated strawberries once they are six to nine months old. I like to recommend offering small servings of pureed strawberry, such as in a strawberry banana yogurt smoothie or even strawberry ice cream, as a first step toward the whole berry by nine months of age.

Honey: The reason behind avoiding honey is a good one and advice to be taken seriously. Honey can contain spores of a toxin called botulism, which are not a problem for older kids and grown-ups, as our digestive tracts are mature enough to protect us from them. The ten-month-old still has a relatively immature digestive tract and can absorb these spores, making them quite ill. Many parents ask if it is OK to feed their baby foods with honey as an ingredient and the answer is no because botulism spores are heat-resistant. So, to be safe, wait until the twelve-month mark to start giving foods with honey—and begin with something that might be processed with honey, like a cereal.

Citrus fruits: Well known for being "acidic," many parents shy away from giving citrus fruits to babies and young toddlers. It is prudent to use caution with introducing them before six months of age, and citrus also might be aggravating to a toddler who has or is outgrowing gastroesophageal reflux disease. That being said, the twelve-month-old toddler can easily incorporate citrus foods into her diet without any worry. Start with a small serving and offer alone for the first few times to make sure she does not have a reaction.

Wheat: Research has shown that delaying the introduction of wheat into an infant's diet after seven months of age or offering wheat before four months of age may increase the risk of developing wheat allergy, celiac disease, and possibly type 1 diabetes. Once your infant has turned seven months, it is important to incorporate basic carbohydrates such as whole wheat breads, oats, or even barley as the latter two foods listed are often contaminated with wheat flour. This will provide an exposure to wheat in one form or another.

Choking hazards

Unfortunately, many toddlers spend their mealtimes... well, toddling around, with food in hand eating on the go. Generally speaking, one- to three-year-olds don't have any interest in sitting down for prolonged periods of time, and desperate parents will hand them some food to finish as they slide off their seat at the table (I confess, I am guilty of this too). However, it is important to know that this is not only undermining any efforts you have made toward keeping your toddler at the table eating, but also can put your toddler at risk of choking. Here are some ground rules to prevent a choking episode:

1. Insist that kids sit when they eat.

2. Do not allow toddlers to eat foods in the car; if they were to choke on something while you are driving, it would be very difficult (not to mention dangerous) to help them.

3. Offer foods in small bite-sized pieces—about the size of your pinky fingernail for the twelve- to twenty-month-old, and no bigger than your thumbnail for two years and up.

4. Apply only thin layers of flavored spreads such as cream cheese and nut butters, as these foods can stick to the roof of a mouth, making it difficult to swallow.

The foods listed in the table below pose the highest risk of choking in a toddler—and really apply to kids through age four:

CHOKING HAZARDS
Chunks of meat
Nuts

CHOKING HAZARDS
Hard candies (or other sticky, chewy candy such as taffy or caramel)
Teething biscuits: I often tell families to let their toddler gnaw on a frozen mini-bagel instead of teething biscuits, as teething biscuits can become soft and break apart, leaving a chunk stuck in your toddler's throat.
Raw vegetables (carrots, celery, peppers, cucumbers)
Fresh fruits in large pieces (apples, grapes, orange segments, pineapple, melon in large chunks or balls)
Popcorn (stick with Pirate's Booty or Nude Food)
Hot dogs, sausages, kielbasa (hot dogs need to be cut down the middle, and then each half needs to be cut again before cutting horizontally).

Do teeth really matter?

I think one of the most frequent comments I hear from parents is that they delay offering meats because their one-year-old doesn't have any teeth, and they don't "want her to choke." Although it is entirely true that chunks of meat can cause choking in a child with or without teeth, small pieces of softer cooked meats such as a small meatball, meatloaf cut into quarters, or shredded pieces of baked chicken, fish, or turkey would not. More importantly, your toddler doesn't really need teeth to chew—in fact, toddlers will learn to "gum" food to a pulp just fine.

The most important thing you can do to minimize the risk of choking is to be sure kids are seated safely at a table supervised by you the parent, and foods are offered in small manageable pieces (starting with the size of your pinky fingernail). If you are concerned about your one-year-old's ability to safely eat nutritious foods like fresh fruits, you can try using the mesh Baby Safe Feeder (www.babysafefeeder.com) to help your toddler eat safely.

Moving to table foods: expanding your toddler's diet

In chapter one, we talked about how to expand the number of foods your toddler is eating by identifying the types and textures your tot enjoys. This chapter will build on food exposure by introducing you to the concept of REAP: role-model, expose, amplify, and plan to *reap* the benefits of eating proper and wholesome food. So what exactly does REAP mean?

Role-model: You and your husband (partner) eat these foods often yourself.

Expose: You serve these foods often (for example, two to three times per week).

Amplify: You put some real effort into making these foods taste good by enhancing their flavor.

Plan and Present: You serve them in a favorable, non-threatening way with a food your toddler already accepts, ideally when he is especially hungry.

ROLE-MODEL

Parents hold a large amount of power to help encourage toddlers to try new foods. Simply by sitting and eating the same foods as he is in front of him, you are role-modeling "good" eating habits, which over time can leave your toddler wanting to "do as you do." I have a very fond memory of a family who came to my office on a recommendation from their pediatrician. Baby Tyler had to eliminate milk from his diet early on as an infant, but now as a twenty-month-old, he had successfully reintroduced milk back into his diet and was thriving. The doctor just wanted his parents to "check in" with a registered dietitian to make sure Tyler's diet was advancing appropriately for his age and to allow his parents to ask any pressing questions about nutrition they might have. As it turns out, I was the one asking the most questions.

Tyler was happy, growing along his own curve, and ate everything under the sun. I mean everything: shellfish, wild rice, lamb, steak, salmon burgers, casseroles—the list went on. I could not name a food he had not tried, which is not a typical event in my office. You see, I spend most of my days helping parents *find* foods their toddler will actually *eat*. Tyler's parents sensed my bewilderment—so I had to ask: How did you do it? How do you get him to eat all of those foods? They both chuckled and straightforwardly replied, "We feed him what we eat." They went on to explain that the house rule for all three of their children was to find something to eat on the family table. No exceptions. Both admitted that there were always some meals favored more than others, but overall there is minimal fuss because they as parents set a consistent example each night.

It was an "Allelujah!" moment for me as a dietitian, proving over fifty years of research on feeding behaviors and parental influence to be tried and true.

EXPOSE

Consistent exposure or introduction to a new food is one of the best ways to avoid struggles with toddlers. You should offer a new food at least once per week to keep momentum going and remember that it can take an average of nine to fifteen times for your toddler to see it before she might even touch it. Let's look at an example for the best approach on offering a new food.

How to offer a new food

Typical approach: New food: mango, offered as snack

TODDLER: What is it?

PARENT: It's mango. *(take a bite yourself)* It's delicious.

TODDLER: I don't like it! *(shoves bowl away)*

PARENT: How do you know? You've never had it.

TODDLER: I want diced peaches. I don't like mango.

PARENT: We don't have any diced peaches. We have mango.

TODDLER: *(crying)* But I want peaches!!!

PARENT: *(sweating)* Eat the mango—it's good for you; you'll like it—it tastes just like peaches. Just take a bite.

TODDLER: *(through clenched teeth)* I want peaches!!!! *(runs from the table)*

Best approach: New food: mango, offered as part of a meal along with a safety food.

TODDLER: What is it?

PARENT: Fruit.

TODDLER: I like fruit.

PARENT: Me too. *(takes a bite)*

TODDLER: *(may or may not take a bite but remains at the table; touching the fruit would be a big step toward acceptance)*

Use this technique any time you introduce a new food—at least once a week.

AMPLIFY

Remember in the beginning of this chapter when we were comparing packaged food to homemade food and I asked you, "What would you rather eat?" Nobody would argue that they would rather eat food that tastes good. For toddlers, taste is everything when it comes to food acceptance. Amplify means to take the foods you are serving and make them full of flavor. The secret is to add a little bit of seasoning and fat for a lot of flavor. So the next time you are making steamed carrots, add a dab of butter and either cinnamon or a pinch of salt to make them extra yummy. Or add a spoon of cream cheese and diced chives to your next omelet.

Michael's Story

Three-year-old Michael was the only child to a working single mother of advanced maternal age (forty-two); he had suffered from food allergies up until he was two, and was now coming to our office for weight loss. Michael's mom had been so overwhelmed as a single parent of an allergic child that she never really had time to learn about basic nutrition and feeding. Most of her effort was put into learning what foods to avoid, how to read a food label, and how to use an EpiPen for the first year of his life. So, when Michael's food allergist told her he had outgrown his food allergies to soy, milk, and eggs, she was unprepared to move forward and feed him as a "normal" child, without any dietary restrictions.

As we sat together in my office, I learned that she had trained herself to make things as plain as possible

TODDLER-FRIENDLY FLAVORS

Sweet and savory: cinnamon, nutmeg, allspice, brown sugar, ricotta cheese

Tart and tasty: orange juice, fresh squeezed lemon, lime, or tomato juice

Robust and rich: garlic, basil, "steak seasonings," cumin, dried mustard powder, sharp cheddar cheese

because she was afraid of Michael having a reaction to food: plain boiled pasta, boiled potatoes, baked meats with minimal seasoning, and vegetables without any added fat (oil or butter). This pattern continued despite knowing that Michael was now cleared by the doctor to eat anything. We had a discussion on basic cooking, adding flavor with different fats, seasonings, and a small amount of salt.

When Michael came back to the clinic after a few months, he had started to gain weight. He and his mom were for the most part eating the same meals now, and it was clear that she had really needed some time to relax a bit about food—and believe for herself that Michael was going to be safe after eating foods he was once allergic to.

PLAN AND PRESENT

Having a plan for your meals each week will help you stick with a feeding schedule and stay true to your goals of presenting a new food. For example, if you have found that on too many occasions you plan to serve say, lasagna, but bail at the last minute and just give your toddler something you know he will eat such as chicken nuggets, then you need to focus your effort on having a weekly menu—and stick to it. Ideally, you should plan a *two-week cycle menu* and make sure some dishes are reappearing frequently enough to jog your toddler's memory. This will help him become familiar and comfortable with the new foods. See the following chart for more information on planning a cycle menu.

Presenting food (new or not) can be difficult for parents of toddlers. In order to REAP the benefits of new foods, you must force yourself to avoid asking the dreaded "What do you want for lunch?" Most toddlers have no clue what they want to eat, and will often blurt out what might be most familiar, or simply try and please you by providing an answer to your question. Asking a toddler is a tricky trap because ultimately, you are relinquishing all of the control over mealtime. And even if you serve him what he asks, he might decide not to eat much of it to see what else he can control.

You as the parent know what is best for breakfast, lunch, and dinner—not your toddler. My colleague Beth told me when her kids were little, they would say,

"What's for dinner?" and she would always proudly tell them exactly what was for dinner: "Breaded chicken, sautéed spinach, and roasted potatoes." Almost always, someone would gripe about something, so since then she has answered that same question with one simple word: "Food."

THE CYCLE MENU

	MONDAY	TUESDAY	WEDNESDAY
Week 1	Breaded chicken cutlets Green beans Baked potato	Spaghetti and meatballs Broccoli Garlic bread	Grilled cheese Tomato soup with Goldfish swimmers
Week 2	Penne and broccoli Chicken sausage	Turkey tacos Yellow rice Peas and corn	Shepherd's pie Applesauce
Repeat Week 1 (use main meal with a slight variation)	Breaded chicken tenders with fresh-squeezed lemon	Spaghetti and meatballs (try chicken meatballs)	Grilled Black Forest ham and cheese

WHAT IS A CYCLE MENU?

A cycle menu is a menu that repeats itself at the end of the two-week period. You can make a menu for any time period (e.g., two to four weeks), and then after the two weeks is over (or whatever time period you choose), you

THE CYCLE MENU

THURSDAY	FRIDAY	SATURDAY	SUNDAY
Cheese ravioli Cooked peas and carrots	Pizza—take out Sliced cucumbers, peppers, tomatoes	Grilled flank steak Rice Corn Fresh fruit	Oven-roasted chicken Mashed sweet potatoes Mixed vegetables
Apple and cheese quesadilla Sliced peppers	Roasted turkey breast Baked potatoes Salad	Salmon cakes Diced mango Green salad	Soup Warm bread or good crackers
Spinach and cheese ravioli Steamed carrots Ciabatta bread	Pizza or junk food night	Grilled meat or fish Steamed zucchini or yellow squash Confetti rice (brown rice mixed with chicken flavoring)	Oven-roasted chicken or pork tenderloin Mashed Yukon gold potatoes Sautéed green beans

repeat it. Having a planned menu will keep you focused on the long-term goal of expanding your toddler's diet, and in the short term, provide resolution to the ever-challenging conflict of what to make for dinner. Buy a chalkboard for your kitchen and write up the meal of the evening first thing in the morning, so when the day is done and you walk in the door, there are no questions asked. Be sure to plan for "free nights," or what we call "junk-food night," where each member of the family can choose what they would like to eat: something convenient and easy to make that might not be 100 percent nutritious (e.g., frozen pizza or homemade nachos).

For this type of menu to be successful in your home, I always urge parents to plan time to shop for what they need to make the menu a success—and if you can shop sans kids a few times a month, that is ideal.

When planning your menu be sure to include familiar safety foods your toddler will readily accept, even if they are offered as a side dish. When planning my own cycle menu, I often keep the main part of the meal, such as the protein, the same and change up the veggies and carbohydrates with what I have available.

You can see this in the cycle menu in the third row where the menu repeats itself: the blueprint remains the same—chicken, pasta, sandwich, ravioli, junk-food night, grilled meat, oven-roasted meat—however, the variety, side dishes, and flavors vary slightly. You can define your own categories for menus based on foods your family gravitates to. For example, some people include a "vegetarian night" and opt to serve a dinner without any meat. By default, you might already be doing this when you heat up a jar of tomato sauce and boil a box of pasta. Don't feel bad about this—just intend to do it and call it vegetarian night. Be sure to serve a side of broccoli, a fresh green salad, or, even better, both.

The Samela house is forever known for our infamous "chicken cutlet Wednesdays." Neighbors have actually walked right by our house at dinnertime, heading into town to grab a slice of pizza, without asking us to join them because it was Wednesday! I often will use different cultures to influence the flavor of the main part of the meal, such as the chicken cutlet:

- Breaded chicken cutlet + fresh squeezed lemon + a splash of white wine served with angel hair pasta
- Breaded chicken cutlet, sliced into strips + BBQ sauce for dipping + oven-baked fries
- Breaded chicken cutlet + tomato sauce + shake of parmesan cheese + mini rigatoni

PLANNING FOR MEALS OUTSIDE THE HOME

If planning for dinner is half of the battle on what to offer your toddler, then the other half is what to send for lunch if your toddler is attending preschool or day care.

When planning a packed lunch, I often encourage parents to think about the sandwich dissected, and remind them that the sum of the parts is as good as the whole. The sandwich can be your blueprint for planning meals for toddlers. Consider for one moment the store-bought lunch packs, or Lunchable. The Lunchables package is the quintessential toddler meal to go. It has easy-to-pick-up foods, balanced with protein, fruit, and carbohydrates that are precut and packaged in perfectly proportioned sections that don't touch each other. The problem is that some of the packs are highly processed with refined grains and a lot of salt—not exactly something you want to pack for your toddler's school lunch every day. The good news is that these meals can be easily replicated at home by using small, reusable containers or new lunch packs available for kids' meals on the go.

Perception completely applies to menu planning. So what if you make chicken three nights per week? It's how you make it that counts toward building variety: parmesan, quesadillas, breaded, or even as tikka masala!

The sandwich dissected

If your toddler is one of the many that might not be ready for a sandwich, consider that some toddlers will gravitate toward crackers in place of bread, so if your toddler is one of these, aim to offer whole-grain crackers on most days, and on others be sure to keep the image of a tea sandwich in mind—crustless, tiny, and flat with something yummy in between.

Beyond the deli meat

It might not be the bread that your toddler is shying away from when it comes to the sandwich—you also need to consider what you are putting in between. Try one of the following combinations to help your toddler learn to like the sandwich, and be sure to spread it thin:

Whipped cream cheese + jelly (alternating flavors)
Apple butter + peanut butter
Pub cheese + thinly sliced cucumbers without the skin
Baby bruschetta: store-bought olive tapenade mixed with a little cream cheese spread
Hummus + one slice of cheese
Refried beans + one slice of cheese
Nutella + Fluff
Thinly spread chicken salad (made with mayo, without celery)

| Sunflower butter + soy nut butter and honey |
| Muenster or other soft cheese with mustard and mayo blend |

Moving from exposure and planning to Nutrition 101, chapter three will help your toddler REAP the benefits of healthy foods, and help you identify which foods are worth those fifteen exposures due to their nutritional superiority.

Here is a list of bread substitutes if your toddler prefers crunchy over soft and squishy:

3–4 Wheat Thins

1 handful of Pop Chips or small, round multigrain tortilla chips

Whole Grain Ritz, Late July Butter Rounds, Pepperidge Farm butterfly crackers

Veggie Chips or Stix

Rice cakes, all flavors

Mini Stone Wheat Crackers, Trader Joe's Multigrain Crackers

CHAPTER THREE

Nutrition 101

One of the hardest things for the parents of a toddler to understand is that toddlers only need very small quantities of food to grow and thrive. Time and time again in my office, I listen to parents report with exasperation what little their tot has eaten in a day, and empathize with their concerns—it's hard not to feel frustrated for anyone who has sat at the table with a two-year-old pushing peas around his plate or a three-year-old blatantly refusing to try a new dish you have enthusiastically prepared. Because toddlers eat such small amounts of food throughout the day, the ultimate goal for feeding should be to maximize each bite of food, making every morsel count toward calories in the bank for spending toward growth. How do we do this? By offering proper foods that are packed with a nutrient-dense punch.

As a dietitian, I am trained to know how to calculate energy and nutrient needs for growth based on the dietary reference intakes (DRIs). My colleagues and I always laugh about our critical need for a calculator: if we show up to work without one, we might as well go home. The DRIs are a set of guidelines from the Institute of Medicine of the U.S. National Academy of Sciences that allow us to estimate how much of any nutrient a child needs based on her age. In short, we can calculate hard numbers, which gives us a place to start with meal planning. It is important to know the DRIs are recommendations for healthy children, and more complex considerations need to be taken into account when determining how much energy (or any nutrient) a sick child would need for growth.

So what nutrients are the most important for growth at this age and how can we best nourish toddler bodies without getting too frantic? First, let's quickly consider what food is actually made up of—and remind ourselves that we are what we eat. Our toddlers are too.

The macronutrients: Carbohydrates, proteins, and fats are nutrients that provide calories or energy. I know: as grown-ups, hearing the word "calorie" immediately makes us start adding up how many minutes on a treadmill we might need to burn off those calories. However, the operative word in the former sentence is "*grown*-up." Our toddlers are not grown-up and greatly need their calories for total body growth.

The micronutrients: Vitamins and minerals are nutrients required for growth, but in much smaller quantities. The list of micronutrients is long—as many of you might know simply from walking down the supplement aisle at your local CVS. For the toddler, I have identified calcium, vitamin D, vitamin A, zinc, and iron as being the most worthy of discussion, since these vitamins and minerals are so intricately involved in the cycle of growth.

Before we take a detailed look at the key nutrients total body toddler growth requires, let's consider all aspects of what else contributes to physical growth and development—beyond food and nutrients.

Exercise: One of the most overlooked critical contributors to bone mass (strong bones) and in turn long-bone growth (which means getting taller) is physical exercise. Health care professionals spend so much time educating parents about what their child needs to eat to have strong bones; however, not nearly as much time is spent with families discussing the need for daily weight-bearing activity. For the toddler, this simply translates to getting outside and playing every day as much as possible. Carving out time for activities such as riding a tricycle, running, walking a few blocks (or even in the grocery store aisles), climbing, and sliding are just as important as drinking a glass of milk.

Love and nurturing: Parenting is never easy, but providing your toddler with a consistent routine, loving heart, and empathy will help a toddler grow developmentally, and be comfortable and confident with who he is.

THE MACRONUTRIENTS: CARBOHYDRATES

Complex carbohydrates are found in familiar grains such as cereals, rice, bread, pasta, tortillas, couscous, waffles, oats, quinoa, legumes (beans), and amaranth, to name the big ones. Fruits, vegetables, and potatoes also provide a source of carbohydrate. A toddler's diet should contain complex carbohydrates at each meal. Today, many people have embraced a low-carbohydrate diet to help with weight loss; white breads, bagels, and white rice have become taboo in many households—which is totally fine for a grown adult and even teen-agers. However, when you have a toddler living under your roof, a rigid low-carbohydrate diet can lead to trouble with sufficient weight gain, energy, and linear growth (getting taller). I strenuously encourage parents to include a blend of carbohydrates in their toddler's diet—both white and wheat.

Simple carbohydrates, such as sugars, can be found in foods and drinks such as fruit juice, cakes, cookies, pastries, candy, and other desserts. These foods should be found less frequently in a toddler's diet.

Why carbohydrates are essential for toddler growth:

- Carbohydrates provide the body with energy, and not just energy to run around, have tantrums, and do all of the activities toddlers love to do, but energy for actual growth. If you have ever weight-trained, you know that protein from food maintains muscle mass, but carbohydrates are what give you the energy you need to complete three sets of ten repetitions of shoulder presses. Those repetitions are what build mass (or cause growth).

- Carbohydrates are the preferred fuel for the brain; a growing brain especially will get first dibs on the quickest, most readily available form of energy. Since the brain sits at the top of the food chain for life function, in absence of adequate carbohydrate, muscle mass will eventually be broken down for the brain to use as energy (yikes!). Clinically speaking, this is what we call starvation.

- Carbohydrates provide essential B vitamins that play a role in how the body converts food to energy. Basically, the B vitamins turn table food into gas for an empty fuel tank. Fortified grains such as cereals, crackers, and whole-grain breads also contribute to the majority of a toddler's iron, zinc, and folic acid intake, which we will talk more about later on in this chapter.

- Whole-grain carbohydrates provide both soluble and insoluble fiber, critical nutrients to regulate digestion and, well, pooping! The secret is to make sure your toddler is getting a blend of fibers, which means fibers from whole grains (breads, rice, cereals, etc.) and fruits and vegetables. Fiber will be discussed in more detail in chapter seven, which talks about digestive issues of toddlerhood.

- Lastly, from your toddler's perspective, carbohydrates are easy to like (who doesn't like a warm toasted bagel with butter or a bowl of pasta?), which is why they should be offered with every meal to encourage food acceptance. And, from the young toddler's perspective (the twelve- to eighteen-month-old), they always seem to appreciate the soft squishy texture of a pumpkin bread or even a soft tortilla with melted cheese on it. These types of squishy solids do not break apart in the mouth (think rice), nor do they require a lot of chewing (think pizza crust), so they are easy to form into a bolus (which is basically a hunk of food that sticks together in your mouth so you can get it down in one efficient swallow).

Annie's Story

Sweet little Annie was a two-and-a-half-year-old toddler who by default was put on a low carbohydrate diet as a result of her parents dieting for weight loss (which was unknown to me at the beginning of the consultation). Her pediatrician had referred her to our specialty practice when, at a sick visit for an ear infection, he noticed that her weight was down from her two-year well-visit check-up. As we sat in my office together, I listened to what a typical day was for Annie, with regard to eating.

Most of her carbohydrate sources were from fruits and vegetables, but she was lacking complex grains to provide her with a good source of energy and B vitamins. For breakfast she ate mostly eggs with some melon or occasional oatmeal; lunch was vegetable soup with a mozzarella cheese stick and some fruit; afternoon snack was slices of ham or turkey rolled up; and dinner consisted of grilled/baked chicken or fish with steamed vegetables. At two years old, Annie's mom changed her from whole milk to one percent upon instruction from her pediatrician, of which she drank about sixteen ounces per day and took a multivitamin with iron.

Mom was worried about her lack of energy and described Annie as being "cranky" all the time. When asked how long Annie had been eating a low-carb diet, Mom looked surprised. She went on to explain that she and her husband had been following this diet with great success (kudos to both!) for about eight months—and never even thought it was unhealthy for her daughter, since they both had lost weight and felt so much better since making the change. I reassured her that the foods Annie was being offered were healthy and could be kept in her diet—then went on to explain that Annie simply needed a "carbo-boost" at each mealtime to give her the energy she desperately needed for growth and to play. We discussed adding one carbohydrate at each meal (white potato, sweet potato, buttered pasta noodles, whole wheat bread, or white or brown rice) and offering seconds of the carbohydrate if Annie requested it. I stressed that serving a mix of white and whole-wheat carbohydrates was perfectly fine to keep Annie interested. In addition, because Annie was actually losing weight, we changed her milk back to whole milk and made sure she had some olive oil, canola oil, or butter added to her veggies, pasta, and potatoes.

At Annie's next follow-up visit, she had started to regain her weight and was enjoying the new additions to her diet. Since her mom was keeping up with the carbohydrates and added fat, we opted to switch her from whole to 2 percent milk. Although less frequently, Annie was still cranky from time to time, but her mom came to the conclusion that it was just part of being two!

BEST CARBOHYDRATE CHOICES FOR TODDLERS

CARBOHYDRATE	VARIETY	HOW TO SERVE
Soft-cooked pasta	Penne, ziti, rigatoni, mezzi rigatoni, ditalini, orecchiette (little ears)	Butter, olive oil, parmesan cheese, 1–2 spoons of tomato sauce or pesto
Soft whole-grain breads	Freihofer's Stone Ground 100% Whole Wheat, Arnold 100% Whole Wheat, Wonder Whole Grain Wheat, Arnold Pocket Thins (soft pitas), Milton's Multi-Grain (best toasted with butter), Pepperidge Farm Goldfish, whole wheat sandwich bread	Toasted or not, with butter, jelly, cream cheese, cinnamon, apple butter, or as a sandwich with protein in between

CARBOHYDRATE	VARIETY	HOW TO SERVE
Potatoes	White baking, Yukon Gold, baby reds, sweet, frozen fried	Baked, smashed, grilled, or roasted
Mini-bagels or English muffins	Whole wheat, plain, honey wheat, cinnamon raisin	Toasted with cream cheese, butter, melted cheese, or pizza'ed (add tomato sauce with shredded mozzarella for a pizza twist)
Waffles, pancakes, French toast	Store-bought: Van's Mini Waffles, Eggo Nutri-Grain Honey Oat Waffles, Trader Joe's Banana Waffles, Whole Foods Mini Vanilla Waffles	With butter, maple syrup, Nutella, or powdered sugar and fresh fruit

CARBOHYDRATE	VARIETY	HOW TO SERVE
Muffins and sweet breads	Banana, pumpkin, zucchini, blueberry, bran	Warm plain or with cream cheese, cut into small squares
Brown rice or barley	Long grain, Minute, or basmati; whole pearled (barley)	As a side dish or in soups, such as vegetable or beef barley
Crackers	Whole grain (Wheat Thins, Triscuits, Milton's Whole Wheat Sesame, Carrs Whole Wheat Crackers)	With butter, plain, or with spreadable cheese
Tortilla	Small round, whole wheat, white, or corn	With cheese and refried beans or try with peanut butter and banana

THE MACRONUTRIENTS: PROTEIN

There is no doubt that protein wins the contest for the nutrient receiving the most press over the past decade.

Many may argue that I left out a key word from that sentence and that it should read "for receiving the most *good* press over the past decade." Protein can do no wrong. Everybody is eating it—and a lot of it.

But what role does protein play in a toddler's diet, and do they need as much as we think we do? Let's first take a look at how protein functions in the body. My guess is that I am preaching to the choir, as many of you may already know that the importance of protein in health and nutrition cannot be underestimated. However, one small piece of information has been lost in translation when discussing protein needs—specifically when considering a toddler's diet—and that is quantity.

Protein is essential to human health in that all living cells in our body depend on protein to make things function properly. Food proteins that we eat are made up of amino acids, and once these amino acids are digested and absorbed, they can be used for essential life-sustaining functions. Determining the amount of protein a toddler needs in a day is complex, as it depends not only on the *quantity* of protein consumed, but also the *quality* of protein. In addition, how protein is used by the body will depend greatly on the amount of carbohydrate and fat in the diet. That is why it is so important to eat a well-balanced diet, inclusive of all macronutrient groups.

So what exactly does quality protein mean?

The quality of protein from food that we eat is

determined by the amino acid pattern as well as the digestibility. For instance, proteins derived from animals, like milk protein, egg protein, meat, and fish are considered to be of high biological value because all of the amino acids these foods provide are absorbed at greater than 95 percent and can be readily used by the body. For vegetable proteins such as legumes (beans) and soy-based products, the digestibility (or biological value) is estimated to be at 70 to 80 percent.

QUALITY PROTEINS

Whole eggs

Cow's milk

Cheese

Chicken

Turkey

Pork

Lamb

Beef

Fish

Peanut butter

Beans

Natural soy protein
   (e.g., milk, tofu, yogurt)

This does not mean you have to offer animal-based protein at each meal of the day; however, because we know by now that toddlers thrive on small portions of food, they can get more bang for their buck by eating just half of a scrambled egg versus the "biological" vegetable equivalent of a quarter to a half cup of beans. The best way to be sure your tot is meeting his daily protein needs is to offer a variety of quality protein foods at each meal throughout the day to optimize growth potential.

For the meat-weary toddlers, give at least two opportunities throughout the day to eat meat until they become confident with chewing the texture and begin to accept it on a regular basis.

So what does protein actually do for toddlers?

- Things that happen in our bodies every day, multiple times per day, such as digesting food, blood clotting, muscle contractions, and brain waves are dependent upon enzymes, which are all made from protein.
- Protein can be used as a source of calories that does not influence blood sugar (think calm, focused child) and can promote a feeling of fullness (think happy child).
- Protein helps to maintain lean body mass, which is especially important for a growing body.

How much protein does a typical, healthy toddler really need? The short answer is about sixteen grams per day to prevent deficiency, and a bit more to support rapid periods of growth. But what does that really translate to in food quantities?

One of the most common concerns expressed by parents in my office is how a toddler can eat enough protein in a day when many of them prefer foods other than meat. I often hear parents lament about how many "carbs" their toddler gravitates to and how they blatantly ignore the protein part of the meal. I find myself reassuring parents that meat does take some work—it can be difficult to chew and swallow, and as a texture, it can be hard to get used to. I can't tell you how many times my own daughter, Maggie, would chew on a small piece of steak or chicken and just spit it right back onto her plate (after chewing it for what seemed like hours).

More importantly, I spend a lot of time teaching families that a small amount of protein goes a very long way. Frequently, we ask parents to complete a three-day food record for their toddler when they come to our clinic. This entails writing down everything he eats and drinks in a day, along with any vitamins and minerals he might be taking. When you do the math for grams of protein consumed in a day by a healthy one- to three-year-old, it will always add up to two times more than the recommended dietary allowances (RDAs) for his age. One hundred percent of the time, parents are surprised to learn that their toddler is actually getting enough protein. You might be saying, "Is two times the amount of protein too much?" In most cases of the healthy toddler, the answer is no because these reference intakes are meant to prevent overt clinical nutrition deficiencies. There are no defined intake levels of protein that can result in adverse effects in a healthy toddler; however, if an extremely high protein intake occurred month after month with inadequate fluid intake, dehydration could occur, particularly in warmer climates. Most importantly, if your toddler is tracking appropriately on his growth curve, you have nothing to worry about: he will use the calories provided by the protein as a fuel source for energy.

So many parents over the years have appreciated science-based information when it comes to toddlers meeting protein needs and especially found this information useful when trying to apply the "less is more" concept:

- **Protein is not only found in meat**. Many nonmeat foods contribute to a total day's intake of protein, such as dairy foods (milk, cheese, and yogurt), legumes, nut butters, whole-grain breads, cereals, and pastas. Dairy in the toddler's diet is a big contributor of high biological value protein as it is animal-derived.
- **A bit of high-quality protein goes a long way**. Animal sources of protein (beef, poultry, eggs, fish, and dairy) are considered "high biological value," which basically means the body has no trouble using them—they are ready to go. Ounce for ounce, more protein can be consumed from a tiny amount of meat than a slice of whole-grain bread.
- **The smaller the better**. Tiny pieces of meat are so much more appealing than big chunks. Give yourself a break and start thinking of meat as a side dish on your toddler's plate. As we will explore later in more

detail, your toddler will be meeting her daily protein needs even if she only gobbles up three chicken nuggets and drinks a cup of milk in one day.

- **Think soft and squishy**. Most toddlers appreciate the softer texture of meatballs, meatloaf, slow-cooked chicken, or shredded turkey in gravy over tougher grilled or broiled meats any day.

- **Maximize micronutrients**. Including high-quality proteins in your toddler's diet will give him not only the most absorbable form of protein as discussed above, but also the most absorbable amounts of vitamin B12, iron, and zinc, nutrients naturally found in foods derived from animals and essential for immune and central nervous system function. If your toddler really struggles with meat, you are not alone! Recall our discussion on carbohydrates: many toddlers rely on fortified grains to meet their micronutrient needs. Keep working with meat to help maximize their protein profile while serving up some fortified cereals each morning.

Tommy's Story

Tommy was almost three and driving his parents crazy when it came to eating meat. Night after night they would sit at the dinner table together and watch him eat everything on his plate, except the main course, which was always some kind of meat. His dad was a big meat and potatoes guy, so his mother proudly prepared roasts, steaks, and pork chops each night, pairing them with potatoes and vegetables of some variety. His parents were worried that he was not getting enough protein in his diet, even with his measly attempts at eating tiny bits of meat on occasional nights.

When I asked them to tell me about what Tommy typically ate in a day, it went something like this:

Breakfast: 1 slice of toast with butter, 8 ounces of 2 percent milk, applesauce

Snack: 1 small slice of cheese, 4 crackers

Lunch: 2 pieces of ham rolled up, macaroni and cheese

Snack: 4 ounces of milk and 2 cookies

Dinner: ½ cup of mashed potatoes, green beans, and maybe 1 small bite of steak

Snack before bed: 6 ounces of milk, sliced pears, some Goldfish

Dad made it clear that the "bite" of steak was just that—one small piece. I asked if he ate ham several times a week with his lunch, and the answer was yes. Then I asked if they ever made any other meats that might be softer in consistency, such as meatloaf, meatballs, beef stew, or even pulled pork, and the answer was no.

It was clear I had two goals to meet with Tommy's family:

1. Encourage them to include a few meat dishes that were easier to like, such as the ones mentioned above.

2. Show them how dairy also helped meet his protein needs.

Because his parents were so bothered by his food choices, I decided the only way to *show* them Tommy was indeed meeting his protein needs was to do the math together. So I drew this chart:

FOOD	PROTEIN
Total milk intake	18 g
Ham	14 g
Cheese	4 g
The bite of steak	3 g
1 slice wheat toast	3 g
Total protein intake for the day	**42 g/day**
Tommy's protein needs for the day	16 g/day

Tommy's parents were amazed to learn that he was meeting two and a half times his protein needs for the day (and we did not even count the mac and cheese). They were able to see that about 50 percent of protein needs were being provided by dairy foods (22 g/42 g). I assured them that he was not eating too much protein, as the recommended amount of protein is based on the

DRIs, which are meant to prevent nutritional deficiencies in healthy children.

Next, we went on to make some changes to their dinner menu to expose Tommy to a variety of meats with hopes to expand his palate and improve his overall acceptance of meats. While Tommy was doing fine with what he was currently eating, I explained that having a mixture of meats in his diet would help him keep up his iron-rich protein intake as milk is essentially void of iron. We came to a consensus that three times per week, Tommy's mom would make spaghetti and meatballs with sausage (for Dad!), chicken pot pie, and beef ravioli—both of which his dad actually liked, with hopes that after enough exposures, Tommy would come to enjoy these softer meats on a regular basis.

At the end of the visit, both of his parents thanked me for writing the chart with them—they felt they had concrete evidence to help squelch their frustrations at dinnertime and were excited to finally enjoy a meal together.

After a few months went by, I did run into Tommy's mom at our clinic—they had come back for a final check-in with our nurse practitioner, and Tommy was being discharged from the practice since he was doing so well. I took the opportunity to ask Mom how the suggestions worked out with trying some soft-texture meats. She chuckled a bit and went on to explain that he loved the beef ravioli and meatballs (why hadn't she thought of this sooner? she said), but had not taken to the chicken pot pie. Overall, everyone was satisfied at dinnertime and, more importantly, had settled down enough to enjoy sharing a meal together.

BEST TODDLER CHOICES FOR PROTEINS

Start with a soft texture that is not tough and stringy. Here are some good examples:

Meatballs (beef, turkey, chicken, pork)
Lightly breaded chicken cutlets (try using a blend of Italian bread crumbs and panko bread crumbs for a light and airy texture)
Meatloaf (cut into small cubes or made in muffin tins for individual portions)
Roasted chicken shredded into small pieces
Salmon cakes or fish nuggets
Meats from strained soup
Shredded beef stew
Turkey Slop

> After every Thanksgiving for as long as I can remember, my mother, Patsy, always made a dish with leftover turkey that came to be known as "Turkey Slop," or as my brother Chris

and I call it, "The Slop." It was nothing fancy, just simply all the leftover turkey simmered in newly made (or leftover) gravy. To my mother's credit, her gravy is like liquid gold—but the meat just shredded perfectly and melted in your mouth. Till this day, we have all stuck around the Friday after Thanksgiving for "The Slop," and we now are eating it for breakfast! You can mock this with a simple oven-roasted turkey breast any time of the year.

Pulled pork (think crock pot)

Scrambled eggs with cheese

Uncle Rob's Dirty Eggs

My nephews Jaden and Tyson love their dad's rendition of brinner (breakfast for dinner): scrambled eggs with a shake of cinnamon, just like when your French toast leaves that maple syrup and cinnamon dust on your plate, and your scrambled eggs get a hit of it…yummy.

Deviled eggs

Baked frittata

Strained chicken pot pie

Beef or cheese ravioli

Chicken or tuna salad

Nitrate-free breakfast sausages (made from beef, pork, chicken, or turkey)

Skinless, nitrate-free hot dogs

Man, how hot dogs and sausages have come a long way! Have you noticed there are so many options today? I love the protein content and moderate amount of fat in some of the versions of turkey, chicken, and all-beef hot dogs. Check your grocery store for some of these great brands (and be sure to cut the hot dogs and sausages into smaller pieces and remove tough skin to prevent choking):

Applegate Farms Chicken and Apple Chicken Sausage

Wellshire Farms Turkey Maple Sausage

Applegate Farms all-beef nitrate-free hot dogs

Boar's Head all-beef natural hot dogs

Trader Joe's Sweet Apple Chicken Sausages

So what about being vegetarian?

Today, it seems that most grown-ups are on the same page when it comes to eating animal meat: less is more, or, for the more extreme—none is best. When it comes to feeding a toddler, opting to live a vegetarian lifestyle cannot be taken lightly. We have learned so far that meat supplies a concentrated source of protein, rich in essential micronutrients, such as zinc and iron. And we will learn that meat provides essential fats later in this chapter.

Can a toddler consume enough protein in absence of meat? The short answer is yes; with meticulous planning and proper supplementation when necessary, it can be done. However, because vegetarian meal planning can be complicated depending upon the degree of animal-based foods being restricted, I strongly encourage any parents considering a vegetarian lifestyle (especially vegan) to speak candidly with their pediatrician before initiating. Recall that the quality of protein versus quantity of protein is the key for making this a success. For the vegan, which is someone who avoids all foods that come from animals—including dairy and eggs—relying on whole grains, nut butters, legumes, and natural forms of soy products (e.g., soy milk, yogurt, cheese, and tofu) are essential. If your family follows a lacto-ovo (milk- and egg-containing) vegetarian diet, then meeting protein needs can be quite easy. Refer to www.eatright.org for further reading on vegetarian meal planning for children, or pick up one of these great vegetarian cookbooks:

Enchanted Broccoli Forest
Moosewood Restaurant Cooks at Home: Fast and Easy
   Recipes for Any Day
Diet for a Small Planet
Recipes for a Small Planet

THE MACRONUTRIENTS: FAT

As headlines remind us of how unhealthy American eating habits have become, many families have embraced the dietary guidelines from the American Dietetic Association, the American Heart Association, and even the National Cancer Institute, which all recommend low-fat or non-fat meats and dairy. Although this can be a healthful approach to eating for school-age children and teenagers (the prevalence of obesity among children aged six to eleven years increased from 6.5 percent in 1980 to 19.6 percent in 2008, and the prevalence of obesity among adolescents aged twelve to nineteen years increased from 5.0 percent to 18.1 percent), omitting fat or excessively cutting back on fat in a toddler's diet can be downright dangerous.

In the quest to make America fat-free, we've overlooked a basic fundamental association between dietary patterns and human health: the essential need for dietary fat, especially in regard to brain growth. Sixty percent of the brain is composed of fat, by dry weight, and the cells in our body rely on it for proper function. This is critical to the toddler's development, as brain growth continues through the second year of life—so critical that it is the sole reason why the American Academy of Pediatrics (AAP) recommends keeping your toddler on whole milk until he turns two years of age. The AAP recommendation is based on the assumption that by three years of age, the toddler has a wide variety of table foods in his diet that provides enough complementary dietary fat. Specifically, he is compensating with foods high in fat: cheese, yogurt, added fats (think cooking oils, spreads, butter), and beef. Therefore, switching from whole milk to 1 percent around age two is a nonissue.

But do most toddlers actually have enough variety of foods in their diet? And are they really getting enough fat?

BUYER BEWARE?

A number of functional foods on the market today have ingredients added to them that are touted as being beneficial to your health. A classic example of this is the high-protein pasta: different grains such as flaxseed, spelt, and bean flours are used to make the pasta in place of semolina (durum wheat flour). These pastas provide about ten grams of protein in two ounces, whereas regular pasta provides seven grams. Calorie for calorie they are exactly the same, but the high-protein pastas also provide two times the fiber—which your toddler may or may not be able to tolerate every day. If your toddler is eating a vegetarian diet, then these pastas might be a good option a few times per week, but be sure to mix it up with some good old-fashioned Barilla.

Unfortunately, being raised in a fat-phobic generation, toddlers today are not really getting the fat they need. A recent study by Gerber (the Feeding Infants and Toddlers Study, better known at FITS) showed that nearly 23 percent of toddlers aged twelve to twenty-four months did not meet their daily requirements for fat. This is because so many families are buying reduced-fat tub spreads with patented (engineered) oils, using PAM spray or the equivalent, eating only very lean cuts of white meat, tossing egg yolks, and buying fat-free or reduced-fat cheeses and yogurts, all in the name of good health. Toddlers don't have the chance to make up for the fat they are missing from whole milk if all or most of their other sources of fat are manipulated or taken away.

Furthermore, research has shown that chronic calorie restriction (as you would see in a very low-fat diet) early in life impairs the neurological development of an infant or child. There is also growing interest in the role of nutrition in behavior and learning problems, and a link between attention deficit hyperactivity disorder (ADHD) and fat deficiency is being scrutinized. It is undeniably curious from my perspective that with the increasing numbers of children being exposed to a fat-restricted diet over the past fifteen years, the incidence of ADHD has risen to approximately 20 percent of school-age children during this same time frame.

So what does fat do for the toddler?

- Fat contributes significantly to brain growth and helps regulate the central nervous system, which in turn influences brain function, such as memory, attention span, and IQ. For the toddler, fat keeps the brain wired correctly.
- Fat promotes satiety (the feeling of being full). Without fat in their diets, toddlers can start begging for foods before their next mealtime or sometimes right after a snack. Even as adults, we all know we feel better after eating an apple with peanut butter or a slice of cheese than an apple alone.
- Fat influences taste, which is a key factor in food acceptance for toddlers. The ultimate feeding goal during toddlerhood is to expand the diet—this is difficult to do without added fat because it just makes food taste so darn good.
- Fat is essential to help toddlers absorb key vitamins A, E, D, and K. Because these vitamins are "fat soluble," they require food fat to be absorbed and, in turn, used by the body.
- Fat is also a digestive lubricant. In order to poop efficiently, some fat needs to be present to keep things moving correctly.

This might be a shock to hear, but it is necessary for toddlers to maintain up to 40 percent of calories from fat in their diet due to the fact that they eat such small quantities of foods to begin with. In addition, when you restrict fat, you are also restricting access to essential fatty acids, which are fats that must be obtained from food because our bodies can't make them. In essence, a diet that is devoid of vegetable oils and butter can lead to essential fatty acid deficiency and, as a result, poor growth.

THE JURY IS OUT: WHEN "ESSENTIAL" FATS ARE ADDED TO FOODS

Strolling through the supermarket, you can now find pastas, breads, eggs, and even milk that have added "essential" fat, with the products being labeled as "high in omega-3 fatty acids." The jury is still out on essential fats being added to foods: the source and amount of essential fats being added can vary by brands. Therefore, you don't know *what* you are really paying for when you are, in fact, paying more.

Best advice: stick with foods naturally high in essential fats such as meats, fish, nuts, eggs, and a blend of cooking oils: canola, vegetable blends, safflower, walnut, and sunflower oils. And remember that fortified foods often have very small amounts of omega-3 fatty acids added to them and the labels on the food represent quantities to meet adult requirements.

The easiest way to be sure your tot is getting the fat she needs is to stick to the following rule each day: include one to two teaspoons of added fat at each meal to make each bite of food count. This added fat will provide your toddler with a safety net for getting the calories she needs on days that she might not eat all that much. Please note that the teaspoons of added fat are an addition to the fat she will obtain from other foods (e.g., whole milk, reduced-fat milk, cheese, full-fat yogurt, and meats).

Here are a few examples of easy ways to add additional teaspoons of fat to each meal:

Butter: spread on waffles, toast, pancakes, bagels, English muffins, etc.; stirred into hot cereals such as oatmeal, rice, multigrain, or even corn grits. You should even count the butter used to mix a box of mac and cheese. But don't count spray-on butter or tub spreads that are laden in trans-fats! For the record, I think it's best to rotate real butter with softer spreads that are trans-fat-free, such as Land O'Lakes Light Butter with Olive Oil.

Olive, canola, safflower oil: drizzled on veg-etables, pasta, potatoes, or rice. Oils can be stirred into sauces and condiments for dipping.

Cream cheese: spread on breads, muffins, or crackers.

Nut butters (peanut, almond, sunflower, soy nut, Nutella): spread on breads or crackers, or stirred into ice creams.

Avocado: diced and served alone, or pureed and used to dip with veggies, crackers, or pita bread cut into triangles.

Mayonnaise: used for breading meats instead of eggs; spread on a "tea sandwich" with a thin slice of turkey or deli ham; use to mix chicken, egg, or tuna salad or even add to mashed potatoes.

Sour cream: used to make fun dips for veggies, add to mashed potatoes, or stir into mild salsa for a fun spread on tortillas.

Ethan's Story

Ethan was a two-year-old boy who was seen in our office for poor weight gain and failure to thrive. When his parents proceeded to tell me about his typical diet, they never mentioned fat—not in cooking, spread on toast or waffles, or even a sandwich. When I asked if they added fats to his foods, they both winced in horror. They proceeded to tell me that they only use a tablespoon of olive oil when cooking for the family, and everything else was low-fat or fat-free. They did, however, have a very good reason for being on a fat-restricted diet—Dad had heart disease and his doctor had recommended that he follow it strictly. Once we discussed how fat could and should be incorporated into Ethan's diet for his portions of food, Ethan began to gain weight beautifully.

After I explain the role of fat in dietary health from a toddler's perspective, parents always ask, "What about heart disease? Should we be concerned about added fats contributing to heart disease and high cholesterol?" This question is a very good one, as we have all learned that dietary fats may contribute to clogging arteries over time. However, we have since learned that excess saturated fats and more importantly trans-fats are thought to be most responsible for contributing to heart disease and obesity. Trans-fats are the fats that have been processed as "partially hydrogenated oils" and can be found in all sorts of snacks (even reduced-fat products) that have a long shelf life. Saturated fats are found in animal products or coconuts, and though they can be unhealthy in excess, they are really essential for cell function. I caution parents to limit foods made with processed fats and avoid eating too many fried foods—especially at restaurants. Bad fats, such as trans-fats, are out there—everywhere.

THE MICRONUTRIENTS: CALCIUM

Moving from infancy to toddlerhood often causes distress for the parent of a toddler when it comes to quantifying calcium intake. Up until one year of age, your toddler was either drinking breast milk or fortified infant formula that provided him with all of the calcium he needed in a day. Once table food was brought into the picture, questions such as "how does this yogurt tube add up to four ounces of milk or formula?" or "how much calcium is actually in this cheese stick?" start popping into your head, especially for those toddlers who don't take too well to drinking milk from a cup.

Calcium is required to maintain strong bones, support long-bone growth (e.g., bones that make your toddler taller), as well as for muscles to function properly. Even more important to know is that calcium needs must be met each day—meaning the yogurt drink your toddler had two days ago is not making his bones strong today.

Dietary calcium intake is like saving for retirement—the earlier you start making consistent deposits, the better off you will be as you age. Another good thing to keep in mind for your toddler is that calcium is best absorbed and utilized by the body when it comes from dairy-based foods. When talking to parents about calcium, a discussion of vitamin D always quickly follows. Vitamin D today is all the rage. It has come into the forefront of nutritional media for curing all ailments from depression to high blood pressure, allergies, and even cancer—all of which are simply claims still yet to be proven true. However, one thing we have gained from studies on vitamin D is that basically, we are all deficient, and our bodies need vitamin D to help absorb calcium. Hence, the American Academy of Pediatrics' new recommendations for supplementing all babies, whether they are breast-fed or formula-fed, within the first few days of life with 400 IU of vitamin D.

The reason for the strict guidelines on supplementation is that although our bodies can synthesize (make) vitamin D from ultraviolet rays from sunshine exposure, we as parents are armed with sunscreen, spraying, slathering, or squirting every inch of our toddler's little body, which blocks the production of vitamin D. And vitamin D from foods is hard to get. Not to mention that your toddler (or you) would have to drink a quart of milk (or infant formula) per day to meet the 400 IU recommendation. So what can we eat, besides cow's milk, that has vitamin D? Fatty fish (think salmon), tuna fish, eggs fortified with vitamin D, and fortified cereals. Considering the small quantities of foods we know our toddlers eat, giving a daily multivitamin is the best way to ensure she meets her needs for vitamin D. Specific recommendations for vitamin and mineral supplements are discussed in chapter five.

New 2009 guidelines from the National Institute of Health (NIH) recommend that toddlers age one to three receive 700 mg of calcium per day. Keep in mind that the estimated average requirement (EAR) for the one- to three-year-old is 500 mg of calcium per day. This amount will meet the needs of half of healthy individuals in the age group, so don't panic if every day doesn't add up to calcium perfection. You have some wiggle room (toot-toot, chugga, chugga!).

What does 700 mg of calcium look like in food?

The following food combinations are meant to give a visual as to what 700 mg looks like. It is very important to stress that you should not, in any way, use these guidelines to restrict the amount of food your toddler is receiving, if your toddler is already eating as much or more of the servings listed below. These guidelines are meant to give you peace of mind when some days are not as great as others.

This is what 700 mg of calcium looks like:

2 cups milk (8 ounces each) + ¼ cup broccoli with a sprinkle of parmesan cheese	2 ½ cups milk (20 ounces of milk)
1 YoBaby, YoToddler, or YoKids Greek yogurt + 1 slice deli cheese + 4 ounces milk	1 yogurt tube + 1 slice Swiss cheese + 1 cup milk
1 Dan-o-nino yogurt + 1 cup milk	2 cheddar cheese sticks + 1 cup milk

1 (4-ounce) Wallaby Organic Joey Yogurt + 1 cup calcium-fortified OJ + 1 cheddar string cheese	½ slice pizza + 1 cup calcium-fortified OJ + 2 Mini-Babybel cheeses
1 cup mac and cheese + 8 ounces milk + 1 yogurt tube	1 slice cheddar cheese + 1 bowl cereal with ¼ cup milk + 1 cup calcium-fortified OJ
½ cup ice cream + 1 cup milk + 4 pieces broccoli	1 YoBaby Whole Milk Drinkable Yogurt + 1 slice American cheese
1 Earth's Best Organic Fruit Smoothie + ½ cup pudding + 1 cup milk	1 Laughing Cow cheese + 6 ounces milk + 1 pizza bagel made with 1 slice mozzarella cheese and a side of broccoli

You can see that the list above is loaded with dairy foods. Often parents ask me what nondairy foods have calcium in them. Check below to get an idea of where you can find calcium outside of dairy:

Fortified oatmeal, 1 cup: 350 mg
½ cup firm tofu processed with calcium salt: 250 mg
1 cup cooked broccoli: 70 mg
1 cup cooked kale: 95 mg
1 cup pinto beans: 100 mg
¾ cup fortified cereal: 90–100 mg

Soy milk fortified with calcium: 200–300 mg

1 fortified toaster waffle: 100 mg

¼ cup almonds (use finely ground and add to oatmeal or homemade cookies to avoid choking): 95 mg

1 cup bok choy: 75 mg

3 ounces pink salmon, canned with bones: 180 mg

4 ounces ZenSoy pudding: 150 mg

THE MICRONUTRIENTS: IRON

Iron is a vitally important mineral that is essential for carrying oxygen to tissues in the body—if you lack iron from foods, you can feel tired, look pale, and even become irritable. Iron is always a concern for toddlers because a lot changes from infancy to toddlerhood in regard to dietary iron intake. Roughly one-third of an infant's iron needs are supplied by iron-fortified infant formula or breast milk through six months of age, with recommendations for supplementing iron in exclusively breast-fed babies by four months of age. The AAP estimates that iron deficiency occurs in about 9 percent of toddlers. As toddlers begin to replace liquids with table food, their picky eating habits can leave them at a high risk for developing iron deficiencies. Here's why:

- Toddlers are no longer drinking primarily a liquid diet of iron-fortified formula. Cow's milk, what one-year-olds will start drinking soon after their first birthday, is a very poor source of iron.

- Growth! As toddlers grow, their bodies require dietary iron to replenish stored iron used for growth.
- Toddlers who were breast-fed through the first year of life are frequently prescribed an iron supplement at four months, which parents may or may not continue after six months of age once foods are introduced, despite being unsure if iron needs are being completely met.
- By the time they reach nine months, many toddlers have lost the taste for iron-rich infant cereal, which supplied about 45 percent of daily needs as an infant in just four tablespoons.

Like protein, dietary iron is mostly found in foods that come from animals. This type of iron, which is called heme iron, is absorbed better than any other form of iron from food. Iron that is found in fortified cereals or breads is called non-heme iron, which is the kind of iron toddlers get the most of: breads, cereal, waffles, pancakes, pasta, and even some cereal bars. Though animal protein is better absorbed, we have to recognize and recall that toddlers gravitate toward carbohydrates; therefore, we need to use this knowledge and be sure to provide good sources of likeable, fortified grains every day to keep up with the growing body's demand for iron.

How much iron does my toddler actually need in a day?

The daily iron requirement for toddlers ages one to three is 7 mg/day—this doesn't seem like a big number, but believe me when I say it can be a challenge for a picky eater.

FOOD	MILLIGRAMS OF IRON
1 medium-size beef meatball	2 mg
4 small pieces of meatloaf made with beef (cubes)	1.8 mg
2 slices all natural deli roast beef (Boar's Head)	1.8 mg
2 small pieces of roasted chicken breast	0.5 mg
2 chicken nuggets	1 mg
Fortified cereals (per ¾ cup)	Cheerios: 8 mg Life: 9 mg Cream of Wheat: 9 mg Cascadian Farm Clifford Crunch: 5.4 mg/cup
Fortified instant oatmeal (1 packet)	9.2 mg
Old-fashioned oatmeal (¾ cup dry)	1.8 mg
1 slice whole-wheat bread	0.9–1.8 mg
Earth's Best Vanilla Letter Cookies (9 pieces)	3.6 mg

FOOD	MILLIGRAMS OF IRON
1 Earth's Best Sunny Days Cereal Bar	4.5 mg
Earth's Best Crunchin' Grahams Honey Sticks	4.5 mg
Healthy Times Teddy Puffs	4.5 mg
1 Nutri-Grain Cereal Bar	1.8 mg
Fresh spinach (½ cup cooked)	3.2 mg
1 breakfast sausage	0.75 mg
1 egg	0.7 mg
½ cup cooked beans	2–2.5 mg
1 cup cooked macaroni and cheese	0.7 mg
1 frozen waffle	2.4 mg
½ cup raisins	1.6 mg
1 fig bar (Barbara's Bakery)	0.7 mg
1 tablespoon blackstrap molasses	3.5 mg
½ cup enriched rice, cooked	1.4 mg
1 ounce pretzels	1.2 mg
½ cup cooked green beans	0.8 mg
1 fig bar (Barbara's Bakery)	0.7 mg
1 tablespoon blackstrap molasses	3.5 mg
½ cup enriched rice, cooked	1.4 mg
1 ounce pretzels	1.2 mg
½ cup cooked green beans	0.8 mg

As you can see from the table above, the quantity of food your notoriously picky toddler has to eat to meet his daily iron requirements can prove to be difficult. Making a conscious effort as the parent to purchase foods that are good sources of iron is imperative for successful iron intake.

So what can you do to maximize iron intake?

1. Start the day with a bowl of fortified cereal. Fortified cereals have iron added to them as powdered iron (or "reduced iron"). Check the nutrition label on your box of cereal to find out how much iron is added to the product. Ideally, iron should be fortified at 20 to 45 percent of the recommended dietary allowance. If your toddler likes hot cereals, mix wheat germ into it to maximize the iron content. Or try to offer a high-iron cereal bar in its place.

2. Offer two meals a day that each provide a small amount of meat to ensure the most absorbable form of iron is available.

3. Buy whole grains: ounce for ounce you will get more iron from grains that have been fortified than refined white-flour grains.

4. Use cereal or cereal bars as a snack and offer in the afternoon between lunch and dinner. Be aware though that many of the new organic and "all natural" varieties of cereal do not consistently contain the same amount of iron as your basic Cheerio does—they are usually fortified with less iron.

5. Give a blast of vitamin C at meals: vitamin C enhances iron absorption, so one thing parents can do is make sure when our toddlers are eating meats, they are also consuming an excellent source of vitamin C at the same time. I always like to have fruit on the table with meals, and of course tomato sauce (excellent source of vitamin C) with my meatballs. Try these other good sources of vitamin C:
   a. Kiwi
   b. Potatoes
   c. Tomatoes
   d. Cauliflower (aka: white broccoli)
   e. Broccoli
   f. Oranges, tangerines, clementines, or orange juice
   g. Mango
   h. Strawberries
   i. Fruit juice (4 ounces)—especially cranberry
   j. Cantaloupe
   k. Watermelon
   l. Pineapple

TOO MUCH MILK?

If your toddler consumes large quantities of milk or soy milk, such as 24 to 32 ounces or more a day, with very little food to complement the milk intake, he or she might be at risk for iron-deficiency anemia. As mentioned previously, milk is a very poor source of iron, and too much is simply not a good thing. Talk with your pediatrician if you feel your toddler is simply not eating enough table food and drinking milk till the cows come home.

Iron supplements

Sometimes an iron supplement is necessary, despite supermom efforts at including good sources of iron at each meal. If you have been told your toddler still needs an iron supplement, and all other causes of iron deficiency have been ruled out, don't feel bad. At times, foods high in iron just don't cut it for keeping up with demands of the growing body. Supplements are needed in this circumstance because it is simply too risky to rely on just food intake to correct a deficiency, since the amount of food a toddler eats every day is so variable. Rest assured, most situations do not require long-term supplementation; it is simply done to put your toddler back on track. And it is not your fault as a parent.

When I was told my daughter Maggie needed an

iron supplement at her one-year well-visit check-up
after a routine blood test in the office, I must have
looked like a deer in headlights. Thoughts were racing
through my head, and I could not stop thinking about
what I had done wrong. I mean, she wasn't the *best*
eater, and she did spit out much of the meat we all
tried to feed her through the first year of her life. But
come on! Could this really be happening to me?

My pediatrician picked up on my feelings of guilt and
reassured me that all would be fine if I gave her the
supplement for the next three to four months—and he
was right. At the next appointment, they rechecked her
hemoglobin level, and it was back to normal. I was able
to stop the supplement, and I continued to keep up her
iron from foods.

The truth about iron and constipation

So many parents come into my office and confess they
have not been giving their toddler the iron supplement
that was prescribed because it makes him constipated. As
you will see in chapter seven, which addresses digestive
issues of toddlerhood, toddler constipation is caused by a
number of different things: lack of fiber, very little food
intake, and too little fluids being major players.

Iron supplements *can* be constipating (some kinds
more than others) and typically at high doses—but
often they are not entirely responsible for toddler

constipation. Before pulling the plug on a much-needed supplement, try one of the following interventions to see if it makes constipation a bit better.

1. Give the iron to your toddler at night while he is taking a bath; have him lie back on your arm, and gently drop it to the inside of his cheek so it has nowhere to go but down. By giving the iron at night, you won't be waiting around all day wondering when he is going to poop, and you will be less likely to blame his fussiness on the iron supplement.

2. Split the dose in half, and give it at two different times per day. For example, if your pediatrician has prescribed liquid iron, instead of giving one full dropper at a time, give half in the morning and half at night (0.5 ml two times per day).

3. Talk to your doctor before stopping the supplement altogether. Ask about giving it three times per week instead of daily; this may lead to improved tolerance, and some iron from a supplement is better than nothing, especially if your toddler really needs it.

THE MICRONUTRIENTS: ZINC

I chose to include zinc in this chapter because it does not typically receive the attention it deserves, even though it plays a very relevant role in human growth. Zinc is also a mineral that is found in foods primarily of animal origin and in whole grains (think red meat, seafood, whole-wheat breads) but also is added to foods during fortification (think fortified cereals). Zinc is essential for normal growth as it plays a key role in DNA synthesis and cellular growth and metabolism, and helps to maintain immune function (which is why you may often see zinc in cold lozenges, etc.). Although zinc deficiency is rare in North America, infants who are solely breast-fed through seven to twelve months of life, without proper foods added to their diet, can become deficient in zinc as they enter into toddlerhood. The simplest way to be sure your toddler is getting enough zinc from her diet is to include meat at least once a day at either lunch or dinner. It is important that any family choosing to follow a strict vegetarian diet makes sure their toddler will not require zinc from a multivitamin and mineral supplement, as non-meat sources of zinc are not nearly as well absorbed as zinc from meats.

If your toddler is especially picky when it comes to eating meat, first and foremost don't give up! You have to keep on trying over and over again—remember, exposure is everything. In the meantime, continue to offer fortified grains every day to help meet daily zinc requirements before you go running out to the store to buy a high-dose zinc supplement. High doses of zinc alone that are not part of a children's multivitamin can cause acute stomach pains, diarrhea, and even vomiting, so avoid using these for kids altogether. However, if you feel concerned about the lack of meat in your toddler's diet, starting a children's multivitamin and mineral complex will provide zinc in an amount that is very well tolerated.

CHAPTER FOUR

Milk, Juice, and More

Now that your toddler is taking big steps toward replacing liquid with solid foods, what exactly should and shouldn't your tot be drinking? With the explosion of blended juices on the market—both vegetable and fruit combos, as well as health-food milk alternatives such as rice, soy, and coconut milk—it's hard to know what and how much is really good for your little tike to drink.

How do liquids contribute to your toddler's diet, for better or for worse?

1. Liquids give toddlers a feeling of fullness, and too much can displace necessary nutrients from complex foods, which can lead to a decrease in appetite and possibly a lack of decent weight gain.

2. Liquids, other than water, contribute excess sugar to a toddler's diet. This can lead to tooth decay, cavities, and even unnecessary weight gain.

3. Liquids lack the complete nutrition needed to support growth and development. Even milk is missing

some essential nutrients such as iron, vitamin C, and fat if you are buying reduced-fat milk. Fruit juice provides 100 percent of daily needs of vitamin C, but among other things lacks protein, calcium, and phosphorus—key minerals involved in bone health.

Overall, your toddler should not be drinking more than thirty-two ounces per day of liquids. Sixteen to twenty-four ounces of that should be from milk and the rest from water and a small amount of 100 percent fruit juice. Let's take a look at some of the common beverages toddlers might be drinking.

MILK

One of the most pressing questions parents come into my office asking is: "How much milk should he be drinking in a day?"

To answer that question, you need to have a basic understanding of what milk contributes to a toddler's diet. As mentioned in chapter three, milk provides an excellent source of protein, calcium, and some vitamin D, as well as phosphorus—all important in building strong bones. Milk also contributes major vitamins such as riboflavin, vitamin A, and some vitamin B12—again, very important for growth. In general, the one-year-old will rely more on milk than the three-year-old for calories as she might still be learning to drink from a cup and soothing herself with a bottle—especially at rest time. Ideally, sixteen ounces (or two cups) of milk per day is adequate for the one- to three-year-old with one added serving of dairy from either cheese or yogurt.

Problems can arise when the toddler is drinking large amounts of milk (e.g., more than twenty-four ounces per day) in absence of adequate food intake. Often parents of picky eaters take comfort knowing their toddler is drinking a ton of milk, as it can contribute significantly to his daily calorie intake. I have had so many parents come in to my office saying they are not really worried about their toddler because he "always drinks his milk." While consistently drinking moderate amounts of milk is a good thing in many situations, it can also put toddlers at risk for developing iron-deficiency anemia as discussed in chapter three.

If your toddler happens to be a big milk drinker with very little food in her diet, it is worth attempting to cut back on the quantity of milk being offered in hopes

Don't panic! Many twelve-month-olds will still want to drink more than twenty-four ounces of milk on some days. This is because they are working hard on learning to replace liquid calories with food calories—and it might be easier for some more than others. Make it a goal to work toward an upper limit of twenty-four ounces of milk per day by eighteen months.

of promoting hunger and motivation to try something new. I always recommend parents take a look at what they are doing now, and cut back reasonably from there. Meaning if your toddler is used to drinking a quart of milk per day, it is unreasonable to think you can only give her sixteen ounces. Nothing happens overnight. Taking away milk too quickly from your toddler could reduce her daily calorie and protein intake significantly, leading to weight loss. In addition, she might feel deprived if you become too rigid about milk and might resort to begging, whining, and tantrums to get what she wants. In this situation, nobody wins.

SO WHAT'S A MOM TO DO ABOUT MILK?

I feel perfectly comfortable telling parents of toddlers who are milk guzzlers with a decent variety of food in the diet and who are growing proportionately that it is OK for a toddler to drink up to three cups of milk per day.

But what can you do if your two- or three-year-old is attached to milk like white on rice, and just doesn't seem to want to eat much food? Here are some simple strategies to consider:

1. Just say no. Toddlers need grown-ups to set limits for them. Period. Half the battle of feeding a toddler

has to do with control and discipline—control desired by the toddler, and discipline (limit-setting) by the parent. Many families I work with can get a handle on saying no to snacks before dinner, but for some reason, parents of picky tots harbor a sense of guilt when they say no to milk. A strategy that I have always tried to use in my own house is redirection. When kids come searching for food before dinner, they sense I will say no, so they go with a request for milk. Instead of a definitive "No!" from me, I will say, "Let's have the milk with our dinner—can you see if your new Finn McMissile cup is clean in the dishwasher?" When I sense I am going to be causing an uproar, I will say, "Hey, do you think you can pour the milk all by yourself into the cup and do a taste test?" The taste test is great because most of the time a sip is really good enough—and the rest can go on the table for dinnertime.

2. Say farewell to the sippy cup when you are home. It is so easy for toddlers to get large amounts of liquid from the sippy cup that many families tote around for their convenience. The problem is many are eight ounces or larger, and because of the portability and inability to spill, seem to be dragged around all day with the toddler—allowing open access to liquid whenever he wants. If you haven't already started

to put milk in a small open cup, then now is the time. By age two, toddlers have the ability to hold a small cup independently on their own. You can begin practicing this skill by eighteen months when your tot is sitting at mealtimes. The open top deters you from allowing your toddler to walk around the house with her beverage, and toddlers gain a sense of feeling like a big kid once they are given the green light to hold a big-kid cup. I love IKEA's small, BPA-free cups, and parents even like the idea of using a Dixie Cup dispenser in the kitchen for drinks like milk and water (be sure to recycle!).

3. Offer milk in a four-ounce cup with a snack. If your toddler eats a snack alone and then comes back in thirty minutes asking for milk, then chances are she could have used some more calories. By pairing a half a cup of milk with foods such as crackers (animal, graham) or two small cookies, you are cutting back on milk with a decoy—whereas if you just give her four ounces of milk when she asks for it without any food, she might see the small cup of milk as "not enough," which could lead to a protest.

There are some circumstances where a one-year-old will need to transition from infant formula or breast milk to something other than cow's milk at one year.

1. Allergy

2. Lactose intolerance

3. Vegetarian/vegan lifestyle

4. Parental choice

CHOCOLATE MILK

I can't write a section on milk and not include the most frequently asked question of all time by parents: can I give my toddler chocolate milk? Now, if I were a dentist, I would be quick to answer no and move on. However, from the seat that I sit in each day, the answer is a bit more complicated. Milk is so nutrient-dense—white, brown, or pink for that matter—that it is difficult to tell parents to take away flavored milk when there are much worse things your toddler could be drinking. This is a perfect example of picking your battles. If your toddler will only drink chocolate milk, and I mean only—and all attempts have been made to add just the smallest possible squirt of chocolate syrup to each cup of milk—then don't sweat it. Be sure teeth are brushed regularly, and avoid giving chocolate milk before bedtime.

If your toddler has been diagnosed with an allergy or is lactose intolerant, your pediatrician has probably already provided direction on what to give your tot to drink after his first birthday. However, if you are a parent who has chosen on your own accord not to give your toddler cow's milk for personal reasons, you need to be sure to weigh the risks and the benefits of all available health-food milk alternatives, and be sure to always purchase the milk alternative that is fortified to the highest level.

The market for health-food milk alternatives has grown about 12 percent from 2010–2011 according to the Beverage Marketing Corporation, as grown adults are seeking "healthier" versions of cow's milk. People are trying to avoid hormones and antibiotics in foods

MILK (1 CUP)	CALORIES	PROTEIN
Whole cow's	150	8 g
Rice	120	1 g
Almond	70	5 g
Soy	100–120	6 g
Hemp	100	2 g
Coconut	100	1 g

that are animal-derived, so these nondairy drinks are quite popular today.

While this is fine for an adult, it can be a huge risk for a toddler, who may rely heavily on a liquid-based diet. Health-food milk alternatives have a lower calorie, protein, and fat content. On many of these products, manufacturers have printed a disclaimer: "Not intended for use as an infant formula"; however, the one- to three-year-old is a very vulnerable population that should also be cautious about using milk alternatives in the presence of a very limited, low-fat diet. And depending on the brand of any of these milk alternatives, some might be better than others when it comes to fortification or enrichment with calcium and vitamins A and D. Take a look at the chart below:

FAT	CALCIUM	VITAMINS A & D
8 g	300 mg	A: 10% of RDA D: 25% of RDA
2.5 g	300 mg	Levels vary
2 g	100 mg	Levels vary
3.5 g	300–450 mg	Levels vary
6 g	300 mg	Levels vary
5 g	100 mg	Levels vary

Take a real look at the amount of calcium, fat, and protein in these milks, and then recall our review on nutrition that highlighted the key nutrients necessary for growth. From this table you can see that each kind of milk alternative has its pros and cons, but across the board they are mostly low in fat and protein, with the potential to be dangerously low, depending upon the brand you buy.

You can see how easy it is for your toddler to miss out on the vital nutrients she needs for growth if she is not getting enough fat, calcium, and protein from other food sources.

If your toddler requires a milk alternative, I can't stress enough the importance of being prudent when reading the nutrition label to be sure the one you choose is supplemented to the max with at least 25 percent of the daily value for Vitamin D and 10 percent of the daily value for vitamin A. Talk with your pediatrician or a pediatric registered dietitian (RD) about which product would be safe for your toddler based on the kinds of food he is currently eating.

Connor's Story

Connor was an eighteen-month-old boy seen in our office for failure to thrive. If you recall from chapter one, failure to thrive is a clinical term used to describe an infant or child who falls from his own growth channel in height and weight on the growth chart. He was allergic to milk and nuts, which required him to follow a restrictive diet. He had been seen by an allergist for the management of his food allergies, but was referred to our practice for weight loss. Connor was on a daily multivitamin supplement, liked some meats, and ate potatoes and rice often. He enjoyed a few fruits and vegetables. His mom had been giving him rice milk to drink and he consumed about forty ounces a day. The amount of food he ate on a day to day basis varied highly, so Mom reported that some days he would drink up to fifty ounces of rice milk.

As we discussed Connor's situation further, I learned that he had started the rice milk when he turned fourteen months old, as Mom thought he should no longer be on "infant formula." This instantly explained the weight loss. Rice milk is essentially fat-free and has very little protein in an eight-ounce serving. Because it was the mainstay of his diet for so long, he really suffered from lack of fat and protein to sustain his growth and began to lose body weight. I wrote a prescription for a nutritionally complete formula that is safe for toddlers with multiple food allergies to drink and had Mom add more fats to his diet such as olive and canola oil—both of which are free of any allergens.

Mom called about six weeks later to report that Connor was weighed at his allergist's office and was gaining weight and even grew a bit taller. Connor started using soy milk in his cereal, which has more fat and protein than rice milk, while Mom continued to use rice milk in cooking. In order to allow Connor to get back on track with his weight gain, we planned to keep him on the special formula for a year and then gradually transition to drinking soy milk by age three. Overall, he seemed to feel much better and was even sleeping better at night.

JUICE

Every time I stand in the juice aisle, I get annoyed. To begin with, there is almost an entire aisle in each grocery store dedicated to juice, or juice "drinks," and despite all of my knowledge and training, I still leave wondering which kind, if any, is the best to buy. From the box and the pouch to juice blends, juice and water blends, and fruit drinks (e.g., Hi-C)—it is overwhelming. After analyzing all of my choices, I always seem to come to the following conclusion. It is best not to regularly buy fruit juice, except for calcium-fortified orange juice, and vitamins that you can get from fruit juice should ultimately be obtained from fresh fruits and vegetables.

WHAT IF MY TODDLER WILL ONLY DRINK MILK FROM A BOTTLE?

So many parents come into my office with huge worries about their toddler drinking milk from a bottle. Most will tell me she drinks water and juice from a cup just fine but can't seem to let go of milk in a bottle. Don't feel like a failure if your eighteen- or twenty-two-month-old is still clinging on to the bottle for most or even all of her milk drinking. Stay calm and set a goal: by twenty-four months, your toddler should transition off the bottle entirely. Use colored straws and even on-the-go cartons of milk (e.g., Horizon) to make drinking from something other than a bottle more fun. For many two-year-olds, setting a date can be successful: "Jaden, your birthday is coming up in four days! What kind of cake should we make? And don't forget when you turn two you get a special cup for your milk like your cousin Graham." For some toddlers, giving the bottle to a favorite stuffed animal or baby doll can work like a charm.

We all have heard that putting a baby to bed with a bottle at night can lead to baby-bottle tooth decay. But did you know the same is true for toddlers who sip all day long on milk or juice from a sippy cup or straw? The constant exposure to a sugar-containing beverage can still lead to tooth decay and poor dentition early in life.

So what makes juice so complicated?

SORBITOL

Today, most juice products on the market are fruit juice blends that always start with apple and pear juice as the first ingredients, which when ingested in even moderate amounts can cause stomachaches and diarrhea in some toddlers. The reason behind this is both apple and pear juice contain a high amount of sorbitol, which is a sugar alcohol that cannot be broken down or digested. Sorbitol travels through your system intact and reaches your colon, leading to cramping, bloating, gas, and diarrhea.

DID YOU KNOW?

Gum-chewing on a regular basis can cause the same digestive problems in teenagers and adults: stomachaches, cramping, bloating, gas, and diarrhea—so much so that when sugar-free gum containing sorbitol is eliminated from the diet, stomachaches stop completely.

Many of you might be familiar with seeing sorbitol listed as an ingredient in sugar-free foods such as cookies, candies, Popsicles, or ice cream. Sorbitol is also ubiquitous in sugar-free chewing gums and even the beloved "fruit snack." Both apples and pears as whole fruits contain sorbitol naturally, therefore apple and pear juice contain sorbitol as well—but it is not something you will find on the nutrition label. Eating one apple or pear usually doesn't cause symptoms in people; however, when fruit juice is bottled, a lot of apples are required to yield a four-ounce serving of juice, making the content of sorbitol higher. It takes about four to five medium apples to make one eight-ounce cup! Sorbitol is also the reason why we give our grandparents prune juice for constipation.

EMPTY CALORIES

The biggest challenge for parents today seems to be setting limits with the amount of fruit juice consumed. If every parent abided by the AAP recommendations of allowing four to six ounces per day of 100 percent fruit juice to help toddlers meet their needs of vitamin C, I might not be writing this part of the chapter. Toddlers today are consuming more fruit juice than they actually need, leading to digestive troubles as discussed above. Too much fruit juice can lead to excess consumption of empty calories. Besides vitamin C, most of the fruit juices our tots are consuming are devoid of any other real nutrient required for growth.

Limiting fruit juice consumption seems like a simple task; however, the fruit juice industry has made things difficult by packaging juices in a wide range of serving sizes. Not all juices are created equal. Even if you have the best intentions to limit juice for your toddler to no more than six ounces per day, this can be thwarted in an instant once you pop a straw into a 6.75- or 8-ounce box. This creates two problems: first, the volume of juice consumed fills up their little tummies with empty calories, and second the empty calories in their little tummies make them feel full, leaving little room for nutrient-dense calories.

WHAT CAN YOU DO NOW TO MAKE A CHANGE?

Don't panic if you have a toddler who is hooked on juice. You can start making some changes in his daily routine little by little, which most toddlers won't even notice.

First, be sure that when you buy juice, it states on the label that it is 100 percent fruit juice, which means there has been no sugar or high-fructose corn syrup added to the mix. Second, be sure to buy boxes packed in four- to six-ounce serving sizes, and avoid ones packed in larger sizes altogether.

If your tot is content to have juice packed in her lunch box, try to pack it three times per week instead of every day, replacing it with either water or milk. However, there are some toddlers who don't eat much away from home. If your toddler is one of these children, leave the juice alone and work on cutting back at other mealtimes.

Sometimes it's the draw of the juice box itself that makes cutting back on fruit juice difficult. In this case I recommend using the juice boxes that are half water and half fruit juice blends, such as Motts for Tots, and limiting to one per day. And don't get hooked into buying fruit juices that are made with artificial sweeteners just because they are calorie-free. Artificial sweeteners are two hundred times sweeter than real sugar, leaving your toddler with the impression that things he drinks or eats can taste that sweet. This makes it that much harder to enjoy food and drink in their natural state.

Lastly, start thinking about juice as a treat for special occasions like birthday parties, celebrations, or a long trip to the beach. In the meantime, focus your efforts on offering a variety of fresh fruits daily in place of juices to REAP the benefit of whole fruits, maximizing antioxidants and fiber.

For a fun thirst-quenching drink that satisfies kids of all ages, try the following recipe:

16 ounces fresh brewed caffeine-free iced tea (I like to use the Iced Tea Bags by Lipton and leave a pitcher outside in the sun for a few hours to steep)
1 cup Simply Lemonade
1–2 slices fresh orange (optional)

Blend together; chill, and serve over ice. You can alter the flavor by using different tea blends or by increasing the amount of lemonade to iced tea.

Chronic nonspecific diarrhea of toddlerhood (CNSD)

One of the most frequent referrals we receive in our clinic is for the toddler who is having loose poops, or chronic diarrhea, for no medical reason. Parents often come in complaining that they are having a difficult time potty training their three-year-old or that the toddler has never really had a formed stool. This is what we call chronic non-specific diarrhea of toddlerhood, or CNSD. The diarrhea is not related to an underlying illness and is almost always caused by excess fluid intake—particularly of fruit juice.

Although CNSD is essentially benign and most toddlers are typically growing just fine, it can lead to slow growth and definitely drives parents mad when it comes to potty training.

Marisol's Story

Marisol was a three-year-old girl who came to our office for treatment of her diarrhea. Thankfully, all of her blood work showed she was not sick, but she was still having a ton of trouble with her poops. Her mom told me she went to the bathroom almost three times a day, and her poop was very runny—she almost never had a formed stool. On occasion, it would even leak out the side of her pull-up. Mom was anxious to get her into preschool but knew Marisol would not be able to go if she was not potty-trained.

We started to go over her diet, and Mom reported that she was a good eater: she liked eggs and ham for breakfast, ate soup for lunch that Mom made, and had dinner at night with her family where she ate mostly chicken, rice, and some corn. Her snacks were mostly fruit snacks, and she drank Capri Sun—a lot of it. Marisol drank about three pouches of Capri Sun throughout the day—one with each meal. In addition, she was drinking fruit-flavored water, which contains the artificial sweetener sucralose, at about twelve ounces per day.

I asked her mom if she was a milk drinker, and Mom said they tried to avoid it because she thought it would make the diarrhea worse. We also talked about whole grains and fruits and vegetables, and Mom confessed she stopped offering most fresh fruit and vegetables to Marisol because she so frequently refused them. As a family, they ate mostly white bread and rice and did not eat whole grains regularly.

After explaining to Marisol's mom that her fruit juice intake, total liquid intake, and lack of fiber could be causing her diarrhea, we made a plan to make some small, but necessary, changes to her diet:

1. Cut back the Capri Sun to one pouch per day, and then, after about a week, switch to calcium fortified 100 percent white grape juice (something that Marisol used to enjoy) at one box per day.

2. Limit Marisol's total fluids to no more than thirty-two ounces per day; set a goal for sixteen ounces (two cups) to be from milk, eight ounces (one cup) from the juice, and the rest from plain water.

3. Mom agreed to serve two slices of whole-wheat bread with her soup at lunch and was motivated to start giving her fresh fruits with breakfast and for snack time, and a vegetable at dinner. Mom also planned to mix white and brown rice together and serve it with dinner to increase everybody's intake of whole grains.

4. Mom was worried about being able to take away her fruit snacks, so we decided to make the other changes first, and then try and cut back on the fruit snacks in the next month.

I reassured Mom that the milk would not make her diarrhea worse and encouraged her to buy some yogurt to get the benefits of all of the good bacteria naturally found in yogurt. This would also help Marisol get the calcium she needed in a day.

At her follow-up visit three months later, Marisol was doing much better. She was eating whole-wheat bread, drinking about one cup of milk per day, having yogurt regularly, and even started eating some green vegetables at dinner. Her poops were more formed, and she was going about one to two times per day. They started potty training, and she was having success. Mom admitted that taking out the Capri Sun was harder than she thought, and on occasion, Marisol still drinks it—but only once per day. As for the fruit snacks, Mom stopped buying them altogether, and Marisol didn't even notice!

BEYOND MILK AND JUICE: WHAT ELSE IS THERE?

Parents are always asking about what else they can give their toddler to drink, especially if they are trying to cut back on milk or limit juice consumption. Here is a look at the usual suspects of drinks for toddlers.

Water

It is safe to say that, as adults, our brains are programmed to drink eight glasses of water each day. Our BPA-free water bottles are never empty—we just can't drink enough. This, however, is not true for toddlers. Although water is vital for health, toddlers who drink more than two cups per day might receive less nutrient-dense milk, as well as suffer from loose stools and a decreased appetite as a result of feeling full.

In general, giving your two- to three-year-old eight ounces of water per day, or a little more if it's really hot out, is fine, as long as she is growing and gaining weight at a regular rate.

For the one-year-old, giving too much water can be a risk for water intoxication. This can occur if water is replacing nutrient-dense milk or breast milk. Ideally, the one-year-old should not be drinking more than four to six ounces of water a day to be sure he is getting the nutrients and minerals he needs from milk.

Remember, eating fresh fruits and vegetables counts toward your toddler's water intake, so be sure to offer them regularly.

Sports drinks and vitamin waters

Sports drinks have become all the rage; people of all ages seem to be using sports drinks in place of water every chance they get. Teenagers, who are already known to be poor milk drinkers, have yet another option to choose from for a beverage other than calcium-rich milk. And as far as parents go, many don't think it is such a bad choice when they consider other options such as soda, caffeinated tea or coffee blends, or the dreaded supercharged Red Bull.

Believe it or not, the trendy sports drinks have reached even the little folks. Often they are used like juice and even offered in larger amounts because people have the impression that they are "good for you." Sports drinks contain sugar and electrolytes such as sodium (salt) and potassium (found in potatoes and bananas)—both of which are extremely important for an endurance ath-lete such as Lance Armstrong. Your Saturday morning soccer star can survive with clean water, a handful of gummy bears, and Goldfish! He definitely doesn't need a Gatorade that supplies nine teaspoons of sugar in a twenty-ounce bottle.

Parents will ask if it is OK to give a sports drink to their toddler if she has been sick with a stomach virus or the flu. In this case, I would say sips of a reduced-calorie sports drink throughout the day are fine in addition to water and some Popsicles. In our practice, we recommend "feeding through" a stomach virus to prevent dehydration, weight loss, and undernutrition in toddlers. This means don't be overrestrictive about what you feed your toddler, despite what is coming out of her. Talk with your pediatrician about what your toddler should be drinking if she gets sick—and make sure once she is better, you start giving her nutrient-rich food and milk again.

A quick word about vitamin-enhanced waters: As a rule of thumb, vitamin-enhanced waters should not be given to toddlers on a regular basis. They can contain up to two to three times the recommended amount of vitamin and/or mineral supplementation for even an adult; as most are made with water-soluble vitamins (the ones we pee out and that don't cause toxicity), they can also have herbs added to them, which can be downright dangerous for the toddler. None of these products are regulated by the Food and Drug Administration (FDA); therefore, we have no way of knowing how safe they really are.

Toddler formulas

Many parents struggling with picky eaters feel like they have had a safety net pulled out from underneath them once infant formula has been taken away. Some find comfort in giving their toddler a nutritionally complete toddler formula, so they do not have to worry so much about what their toddler actually eats.

So, what exactly is toddler formula, and would your child benefit from it?

Toddler formula is designed to provide complete nutrition to toddlers up to two years of age. Unlike milk, it is iron-fortified and basically has a daily multivitamin added to it. The amount of calcium and phosphorus is higher than what is found in infant formula but about equal to cow's milk. In general, toddlers don't need formula and will get most of their nutrient needs met with food. I always tell parents to start a multivitamin and try and stick with whole milk and table food instead of using toddler formula. If you are unsure about whether toddler formula could be beneficial for your tot, talk with your pediatrician.

High-calorie nutrition supplements

Some parents contemplate giving their toddler a high-calorie nutritional supplement to replace cow's milk, with hopes that it will help with weight gain. Today, these supplements come in a variety of flavors and are quite palatable. Most are made from milk protein, but some today are even made with soy protein.

Ounce for ounce they provide more calories and overall have more vitamins and minerals, but essentially provide the same amount of protein, calcium, and fat as a cup of whole milk does. While these products are truly beneficial for toddlers and older kids struggling to gain weight for medical reasons, they are not necessary for your everyday picky eater. Here is why:

1. Toddlers need to learn that nutrition comes from food, not a bottled, sweetened beverage that might wind up replacing meals, instead of just milk.

2. Nutrients in a bottle are not the same as nutrients from food. The vitamin and mineral profile might be a bit higher in a supplement, but the added vitamins are just that—without all the phytonutrients and antioxidants found only in healthy, fresh foods. These substances are found in foods such as fresh fruits, vegetables, legumes, and whole grains that work to put up a defense against the body's natural oxidation process or cell damage. Vitamin C, E, and classes of compounds such as polyphenols and flavonoids are antioxidants. Basically, antioxidants and phytonutrients protect your toddler's body from inflammation, which in turn can even prevent chronic disease.

Eating foods that are rich in antioxidants is always better than a synthetic version.

3. They contain more added sugar than a growing, healthy toddler needs.

If you have tried other ways to help your toddler gain weight but find that these supplements are the only solution that really works, then stick with them for the time being and find a registered dietitian to help you make a plan to include high-calorie foods in your toddler's diet.

INCREASING CALORIE INTAKE

Have you tried:

1. Switching to whole milk.

2. Adding two tablespoons of Carnation Instant Breakfast or Ovaltine to a cup of milk.

3. Blending a milkshake at home with whole milk, a banana, one scoop of vanilla ice cream, and a squirt of chocolate syrup.

4. Pouring Stonyfield Farms Super Smoothie, which comes in a ten-ounce bottle, into a cup and saving the rest for the next day. It's much easier than blending, and the smoothie is totally devoid of the dreaded chunks or seeds from the fruit.

5. Try mixing ½ cup of whole milk with ½ cup of high-calorie supplement.

6. Don't forget to recall the tips on adding fats to foods in chapter three!

CHAPTER FIVE

How Much Is Enough?

Feeding is a biological right of parenthood. It is more than choosing what food to feed your child for its nutritional superiority. Feeding is part of socialization. It is a chance to teach manners and an opportunity to share the ups and downs of a day. The act of feeding is a nurturing one and shows kids (and adults) that you care about how they feel.

Feeding a toddler will inevitably lead to frustrations at certain times, but they will pass as long as you have the ability to know how much food is enough for your tot to thrive and grow—and accept that every day will not be nutritionally perfect.

In this chapter, you will learn what I know about food and servings—information that saved me from going bananas when my very own daughter, from the age of one to two, basically recycled one out of every three bites she put in her mouth (food went in, and then came right back out). First, there are some key concepts I ask you to embrace before reading on:

1. It is common for your toddler to eat only one "good"

meal per day, or even every other day. After this chapter, you will feel confident with your understanding of what a good meal looks like.

2. It is more important to look at what your toddler eats over the course of a week, rather than meal by meal or even day by day.

3. Guidelines provided here are not meant to be used to restrict the amount of food you give your toddler. Use these guidelines as ideal "minimums"—so if he eats more, consider it money in the bank. Every toddler is different, and some will eat more than others. Try your best not to compare your toddler to his friends from the park.

4. If your toddler is not gaining weight and you are worried, talk candidly with your pediatrician about an appropriate referral to a specialist, as there might be something more serious going on. It is never normal for a one- to three-year-old to lose weight or stop gaining weight for an extended period of time.

5. Start small! Remember, half of the success of feeding a toddler lies in your parental perception. The portions you serve older siblings (or what older siblings serve themselves) are not anywhere near

equal to the amount of food a toddler eats or needs to eat.

TRICKS OF THE TRADE

Before I had my own children, I did not focus much of my counseling interventions on serving plates, utensils, or even ambiance. Much of the time I spent with families was about my calculator and food portions. Now, let's just say I have been schooled in the use of proper plates and the like to make mealtime more appealing. Even the way you set the table can have a positive impact on how your toddler approaches the dinner table (think name cards with kid-friendly place card holders).

1. Use kid-friendly plates (www.potterybarnkids.com, www.target.com, www.crocodilecreek.com, www.disneystore.com).

2. Use favorable utensils toddlers can hold and manipulate (example: a dessert fork).

3. Be prepared for a mess. Keep paper towels close by for big spills, but resist the urge to wipe your toddler's face after each bite.

4. Consider bringing back the dinner bell. One of

my colleagues Beth told me about this idea, and I thought it was great. Your toddler might just be intrigued by the sound of a ringing bell, and even look forward to it each night.

5. Make some dinner occasions special. Use mealtime to talk about big and small accomplishments or just the high points of each day. My mother always used the Red Plate's "You Are Special Today" plate when it was a birthday, someone won a game, or for hard work that paid off. As these plates are ceramic, you can use them as a place setting for an older sibling—your toddler might just be curious enough to come sit and see what it is all about. The Red Plate is available at www.redplatestore.com.

BE AWARE—THE FOOD JAG

By now, we all know there can be huge variations in what toddlers eat on a day-to-day basis. One day, they seem to eat everything, and the next day, they might just refuse the very same food they were eating gobs of the day before. My advice is to ignore this and avoid making a federal case out of the situation (e.g., "Matthew, you *just* ate this yesterday and told me you loved it!"). Think of it this way: These comments are more of a declaration of independence than a direct protest about the particular food offered. If you can ignore the objection, I guarantee that one of the next times you offer the food, he will take a chance and eat it.

On the other hand, you might have a toddler who decides that mac and cheese is the only food she wants to eat—for breakfast, lunch, and dinner. This is called a food jag: when a toddler will only eat one particular food, meal after meal, and refuse anything else that is put in front of her. If you have ever heard the saying "an ounce of prevention is worth a pound of cure," apply it here. The best way to avoid getting into a food jag is to prevent it from happening. Offer any one particular food *only* every other day. To help survive these situations consider the following advice:

1. Don't panic. This too shall pass. In the meantime, evaluate the food your child is interested in eating for its nutritional value. Does it have some protein, carbohydrate, and fat? Or is it mostly salt, air, and white flour (think cheese puffs or crackers)? If the food falls into the former category, then you don't have to worry; however, if empty-calorie snack foods are all your toddler is eating, then you have some work to do. Think back to the story of Jenny who always wanted cheese puffs for dinner. Give your toddler some of what she craves coupled with proper food at dinnertime and see how it goes.

2. Resist the urge to bribe, beg, or reward with dessert to get your toddler to try something new. This will always backfire. Most often food jags are not about the food; rather, they are more about the toddler's developmental need for control. The toddler innately wants to test his limits to see if he can get what he wants. Developmentally, he is behaving appropriately for his age. Make no fuss about it and appear disinterested in their strike.

3. Avoid labeling your toddler as a picky eater. You don't need me to tell you that toddlers understand much of what we say in front of them. Even more important, try not to say things around your toddler like, "Brian *hates* broccoli. He *only* eats pizza, right, Brian?" When you label your toddler a picky eater, he ultimately will conform and become just that to please you. Instead, try using phrases that positively reflect on his current food choices. For example, saying something like "Brian really likes corn and we're learning to like broccoli" shows your toddler that you are in it together, so to speak, and have great expectations for what's to come. More importantly, your statement demonstrates to him that you believe his choice not to eat broccoli at the present time will most likely change. It takes away the impression that omitting broccoli from the diet

is a final decision. This can help him keep an open mind to green vegetables in general.

GETTING STARTED

Now let's take a minute to recall the major players of nutrition that we discussed in chapter three:

- Protein
- Carbohydrate
- Fat
- Calcium
- Iron
- Zinc

Using these nutrients, we will build nutritionally sound meals for your toddler by his or her age—the one-year-old, the two-year-old, and the three-year-old. Before you skip to the section for your toddler, read below for the blueprint on meal planning at every age.

Pick your proteins: Here I introduce you to the concept of picking your proteins. You will be asked to "pick" your proteins from a given list, and then build the remainder of each meal around that protein with complex carbohydrates (e.g., breads, pasta, rice, cereals), fruits and/or vegetables, and then a dab of fat. I always teach parents to build their meals around the protein source, as it is so essential for total body growth. Training yourself to think of protein first also forces you to offer your toddler the part of the meal she may like the least. It's easy to just skip the protein and go with a bowl of buttered pasta instead. Building protein into two of the three meals a day provides ample opportunities for exposure, which is the best defense against picky eating.

The amount of protein you need to pick *as a starting point for each meal* (from the chart on page 157) will always equal your toddler's age. This is a simple and mindful way to ensure that you are indeed offering your tot enough protein. The amounts of food you will see listed below might seem surprisingly small—don't fret! You can always add more (and should), especially if your toddler asks for it.

For picking purposes, ages will be defined as

The one-year-old: twelve to twenty-three months
The two-year-old: twenty-four to thirty-five months
The three-year-old: thirty-six months to four years

Pick one protein for your one-year-old at each meal.

For example:
BREAKFAST: ½ scrambled egg
LUNCH: 2 tablespoons cottage cheese
DINNER: 1 small fish cake (golf-ball-sized)

Pick two proteins for your two-year-old at each meal:

For example:
BREAKFAST: 1 slice cheddar cheese
LUNCH: ½ golf-ball-sized meatball + ½ cheese stick
DINNER: 2 tablespoons shredded rotisserie chicken

Pick three proteins for your three-year-old at each meal:

For example:
BREAKFAST: 1 tablespoon peanut butter + 2 ounces Greek yogurt
LUNCH: 1 nitrate-free hot dog + 4 tablespoons cooked beans
DINNER: 2 tablespoons ground beef + 6 tablespoons prepared macaroni and cheese

The combinations above provide your toddler with more than 100 percent of the protein he needs in a day, assuming he drinks at least 1 cup (or 8 ounces) of milk or soy milk. Even if he doesn't eat all of the protein offered at each meal, he will still make it up with snacks and the milk he drinks.

What if my toddler doesn't eat all the protein offered at each meal?

Even if your toddler eats half of what you offered at each meal, he is still meeting his daily protein needs, assuming he drinks about twelve ounces of milk per day, is eating whole grains, and has scheduled healthy snacks. Always remember that it is more important to look at what your toddler eats over the course of the week, not meal by meal, or even day by day. Louise Bates Ames, a revered child psychologist from Yale since the late seventies, always told parents of toddlers that one good meal a day is better than three awful ones. This is sound advice that still stands true today.

What if my toddler chooses mostly dairy sources of protein?

This is not uncommon as many toddlers thrive on dairy foods—they simply love the taste. If this is the case for your toddler, don't give up! Always remember when deciding what meat to serve that it has to taste good for your toddler to eat it. The best thing to do for the meat-weary is to offer red meat regularly, even as often as three to four times per week. This may sound alarmingly high for the heart-conscious, but the government food rules that apply to adults simply don't translate to young toddlers. Choose lean cuts of steak such as flank steak, top round, brisket, or stew meat that is simmered to be shredded, and buy grass-fed ground beef often. Pick one meal to offer meat-based protein each day, and move on. She can make up her iron and zinc needs with fortified cereals and grains and even beans while she learns to like meat.

What if my toddler wants more than what I offer him at a meal?

This is fine, and you should oblige him. If he is showing interest (by motioning, grunting, or asking) for more food, then go ahead and give it to him. This is a perfect opportunity to build a trusting relationship around feeding. Remember, these servings are a place to start! Many toddlers will eat much more than this when given the opportunity. Your toddler knows when he is full so you don't have to worry about him overeating. Chances are, if he eats what appears to be "a lot" at one meal, then expect the next one to be less than ideal—and know it's OK.

How do I fit in calcium?

Fitting dairy in at snack time and offering just four ounces of milk with each meal is the best way to make sure your toddler is meeting her calcium needs. Or, if you find your toddler doesn't like to drink milk with every meal, then as a rule of thumb, be sure that one of the proteins you pick for the day is dairy-based (e.g., cheddar cheese, cottage cheese, yogurt, pizza, or cheese ravioli).

If your toddler is not so fond of milk, refer back to chapter three and review "What does 700 mg of calcium look like in food?" to help him meet his needs each day. Or, read further on in chapter five for a complete list of the calcium content of foods.

POINTS TO REMEMBER WHEN PICKING

- Choose whole-grain varieties of breads, cereals, rice, and crackers for most meals, but not all. For a toddler, it is ideal to have a blend of carbohydrates in his diet to optimize food acceptance and therefore diet expansion.
- Rotate lean cuts of meat with full-fat versions to be sure your toddler is receiving a variety of textures and adequate calories and fat. Be sure to offer red meat several times per week to maximize the iron content of your toddler's diet.
- Use fresh fruits and vegetables interchangeably; it is even OK to offer both if your toddler is showing interest for more food.
- Use fats as needed to increase calorie content of a particular meal—especially if your toddler has demonstrated inadequate weight gain.

- Plan for scheduled snacks. Ideally, healthy snack choices should be rotated as follows:
  - Dairy (full fat or reduced fat, not fat-free) + fruit/vegetable
  - Dairy + complex carbohydrate (offer whole-grain choices about half the time)
  - Grain + fruit/vegetable
  - Fun snack

See the list below for healthy snacks that fit the combinations above.

HEALTHY SNACK IDEAS

4 ounces milk + 2 Fig Newtons

4–6-ounce yogurt cup + ½ banana

1 piece deli cheese rolled up with 1 slice deli turkey

Peanut butter and crackers

1 handful baked cheese puffs + 4 cheese cubes (diced)

1 cereal bar + 4 ounces milk

4–5 whole-grain crackers with cream cheese + grapes cut in half

Sliced melon and 1 ham roll-up

1 cheddar cheese stick + pretzel sticks

Pop Chips

1 hard-boiled egg, sliced in half + 4 crackers

Instant oatmeal made with milk

continued on next page...

½ cup frozen yogurt with sprinkles of Fruity Pebbles (for a special treat!)

4 ounces pudding + sliced strawberries

Whole-grain cereal (dry or with milk, yogurt, or pudding)

Hummus and carrot matchsticks or red pepper sticks

Veggie Stix plus Cracker Barrel cheese cuts

Earth's Best Smoothie

Cheese cuts with 1 slice of salami

Pirate Booty or Smart Puffs + 4 ounces vanilla soy milk

Pouch + Cutie Clementines (cut segments in half to prevent choking)

Raisins and dry cereal mixed together—add some Goldfish to the mix

1 whole-grain toaster waffle with cream cheese and strawberry jelly

Fruit salad (mixed slices melon, plus blueberries)

Graham crackers with ricotta cheese and apple butter

Remember, there will always be room to rotate in some fun treats like cookies, ice cream, or even snack chips. It's best to have a variety so your toddler will see all foods as equals. If you never allow them to have some "junk" for snacks, then they will always and only want junk for a snack. Build it into their routine about two to three times a week so they don't go overboard when they get a chance to have some.

PICK PROTEIN	CHOOSE CARBS	ADD FRUITS & VEGGIES	DAB FAT[1]
Pick 1 for 1 Pick 2 for 2 Pick 3 for 3	Choose 1–2 with each meal and at snack time for every age	Choose 1–2 with each meal and offer more at snack time for every age	Choose 3–4/day
½ meatball (golf-ball size)	½ slice bread	2 tablespoons berries	2 tablespoons olives, chopped
1 slice nitrate-free deli meat	¼ cup (4 tablespoons) pasta	2 tablespoons grapes, halved	2 tablespoons avocado
1 tablespoon chopped meat or fish	4 tablespoons barley	2 tablespoons diced strawberries	1 tablespoon cream cheese
½ nitrate-free hot dog	½ mini bagel	2 tablespoons diced kiwi	1 tablespoon sour cream
½ round breakfast sausage patty	½ English muffin	2 tablespoons diced mango	1 tablespoon salad dressing
1 small sausage link	¼ cup brown rice	½ slice cantaloupe	1 tablespoon mayonnaise

1. Fat can be adjusted to help attain calorie goals.

PICK PROTEIN	CHOOSE CARBS	ADD FRUITS & VEGGIES	DAB FAT[1]
Pick 1 for 1 Pick 2 for 2 Pick 3 for 3	Choose 1–2 with each meal and at snack time for every age	Choose 1–2 with each meal and offer more at snack time for every age	Choose 3–4/day
½ slice deli cheese	¼ cup quinoa	½ slice honeydew	1 teaspoon vegetable oil
½ cheddar cheese stick	¼ cup couscous	½ slice watermelon	1 teaspoon canola oil
2 tablespoons cottage cheese	½ piece naan bread	½ banana	1 teaspoon safflower oil
½ tablespoon peanut butter	3–4 crackers	3 tablespoons diced peaches	1 tablespoon butter, spreads
½ egg, cooked	¼ medium muffin	3 tablespoons diced pears	2 tablespoons hummus[2]
4 tablespoons cooked beans	½ waffle, pancake	3 tablespoons diced pineapple	1 teaspoon flaxseed oil

2. *While hummus is often touted as being high in protein, it is mostly fat from oils and tahini, a paste made from sesame seeds. I opted to include hummus under fats, as it is a very healthy food many toddlers will learn to enjoy.*

PICK PROTEIN	CHOOSE CARBS	ADD FRUITS & VEGGIES	DAB FAT[1]
Pick 1 for 1 Pick 2 for 2 Pick 3 for 3	Choose 1–2 with each meal and at snack time for every age	Choose 1–2 with each meal and offer more at snack time for every age	Choose 3–4/day
2 ounces Greek yogurt	½ small tortilla	¼ apple, peeled & cubed	1 tablespoon health spread
1 small fish cake	¼ cup mashed potatoes	4 ounces applesauce	1 teaspoon olive oil
6 tablespoons mac and cheese	5–7 pieces of oven-baked potatoes	2 tablespoons cooked broccoli florets	1 teaspoon walnut oil
¼ cup tofu	10 sweet potato fries	2 tablespoons green peas	1 teaspoon peanut oil
¼ burger	10 Veggie Stix	2 tablespoons corn	1 teaspoon sesame oil
2 chicken nuggets	¼ cup Pirate Booty	2 tablespoons green beans, chopped	1 tablespoon sour cream
2 fish nuggets	½ cereal bar	2 tablespoons diced carrots	

PICK PROTEIN	CHOOSE CARBS	ADD FRUITS & VEGGIES	DAB FAT[1]
Pick 1 for 1 Pick 2 for 2 Pick 3 for 3	Choose 1–2 with each meal and at snack time for every age	Choose 1–2 with each meal and offer more at snack time for every age	Choose 3–4/day
1 chicken finger	¼ cup dry cereal	2 tablespoons mixed veggies (frozen)	
½ cup bean soup	¼ cup cooked oats	2 tablespoons squash, zucchini	
2 tablespoons egg, chicken salad	10 Bunny Grahams	2 tablespoons eggplant, chopped	
4 mini cheese ravioli	6 mini rice cakes	4–5 thin slices of peppers	
2–3 potato and cheese pierogies	8 Pop Chips	4–5 cucumber wheels	
2 tablespoons ricotta cheese	6 Honey Wheat Pretzel Stix	4–5 grape tomatoes, sliced	
2 strips of cheese pizza	2 Fig Newtons	2 tablespoons cauliflower	

ADD ON THE CALCIUM

Offer four ounces of milk at meals three times per day.

Add handfuls of shredded cheese to potatoes, veggies, eggs, or pasta in place of butter.

Choose one meal each day to offer a dairy-based protein (e.g., yogurt for breakfast or grilled cheese with two slices of cheese at lunch).

Pick dairy-based snacks such as cheese and yogurt.

Now, let's get started on meal planning by age and see how much really *is* enough.

THE ONE-YEAR-OLD (TWELVE TO TWENTY-THREE MONTHS)

Developmentally, the twelve-month-old can really still be quite dependent upon an adult to assist her with feeding. Some might not even be mobile until a year and a half, so they are content being captive in a high chair or booster seat with food on their plate to explore, and hopefully eat. If your tot is chewing up meat and decides to push it out of her mouth right back onto her plate, know that she is experimenting with the unknown. Essentially, she is attempting to gain comfort with that particular food (often meat), and will do this many times before she decides to swallow it.

Using the picking chart shown previously, see how easy it is to plan three square meals for your one-year-old:

BREAKFAST	
Pick one protein	½ sausage patty, diced
Choose a carb	¼ cup Cheerios
Add fruit and veggie	2 tablespoons blueberries + ½ banana
Dab fat	Use whole milk, 4–6 ounces
Snack	4–6 ounces whole milk, 8–10 Bunny Grahams

LUNCH	
Pick one protein	½ cheddar cheese stick
Choose a carb	4 whole-grain crackers
Add fruit and veggie	3 tablespoons diced peaches
Dab fat	2 tablespoons avocado, chopped
Offer milk to drink	4 ounces whole milk
Snack	4 ounces yogurt + ¼ pumpkin muffin, cubed

DINNER	
Pick one protein	1 tablespoon chopped chicken
Choose a carb	¼ cup cooked pasta, grated parmesan
Add fruit and veggie	2 tablespoons green peas + 2 slices of pear

DINNER (CONTINUED)	
Dab fat	1 teaspoon olive oil mixed with pasta
Offer milk to drink	4 ounces whole milk

THE TWO-YEAR-OLD (TWENTY-FOUR TO THIRTY-FIVE MONTHS)

Developmentally, the two-year-old is ready to rock and roll. For the most part, he can feed himself independently with his hands, and during the later ages, he becomes competent in using utensils. Some still require assistance with forks, depending upon what you are serving, but can manage quite well. A small open cup is appealing to the two-year-old, as long as he is sitting to drink. All two-year-olds still need most food cut up into small, manageable pieces, primarily to prevent choking.

BREAKFAST	
Pick two proteins	½ scrambled egg + ½ slice of cheese
Choose a carb	1 slice toast
Add fruit and veggie	2 tablespoons strawberries + ½ banana
Dab fat	½ tablespoon cream cheese, spread on toast
Offer milk to drink	4 ounces whole milk
Snack	½ cup dry cereal + apple slices

LUNCH	
Pick two proteins	1 tablespoon peanut butter
Choose a carb	1 English muffin
Add fruit and veggie	3 tablespoons diced pineapple + 4 ounces of applesauce
Dab fat	Use whole milk, 4 ounces
Snack	10–12 Pop Chips + 1 cheese stick

DINNER	
Pick two proteins	1 medium meatball
Choose a carb	1 slice garlic bread
Add fruit and veggie	2 tablespoons cooked broccoli + ½ slice cantaloupe
Dab fat	1 teaspoon oil, added to broccoli
Offer milk to drink	4 ounces whole milk

THE THREE-YEAR-OLD (THIRTY-SIX MONTHS TO FOUR YEARS)

By now, your three-year-old should be in the groove of structured meals and snacks. Tantrums surrounding mealtime by the second half of the third year of life should be minimal. Sometimes, your three-year-old will try and battle at mealtime if things don't go her way (e.g., you are serving something she might not like).

Always remember to appear disinterested and just move on. Three-year-olds know what to expect at mealtimes, and for the most part, come to the table happily and with some curiosity (OK, sometimes still with apprehension!). Your three-year-old can use utensils independently and drink well from a small open cup, even with one hand. By now your three-year-old is even sitting in a regular chair to eat without assistance. Many will kneel on the chair to support their ability to get food into their mouths.

BREAKFAST	
Pick three proteins	6 tablespoons cottage cheese
Choose a carb	1 whole wheat mini bagel, toasted
Add fruit and veggie	2 tablespoons kiwi + 6 cubes watermelon
Dab fat	1–2 teaspoons butter or cream cheese
Offer milk to drink	4 ounces milk (1% or 2%), if your toddler is gaining weight appropriately
Snack	1 cheese stick, 10 grapes (sliced) + ½ cereal bar

LUNCH	
Pick three proteins	3 slices deli ham
Choose a carb	1 small tortilla, warmed
Add fruit and veggie	4 tablespoons grape tomatoes, sliced
Dab fat	2 tablespoons ranch dip, for tomatoes and tortilla
Offer milk to drink	4 ounces 1 or 2% milk, if your toddler is gaining weight appropriately
Snack	1–2 tablespoons of hummus + 4–6 wheat crackers

DINNER	
Pick three proteins	3 fish sticks
Choose a carb	10–15 sweet potato fries
Add fruit and veggie	8 slices cucumber, 2 tablespoons mixed veggies (cooked)
Dab fat	1 tablespoon tartar sauce to dip (mayo-based)
Offer milk to drink	4 ounces milk (1% or 2%), if your toddler is gaining weight appropriately

FOR *EVERY* AGE: WHAT ABOUT THE AFTER-DINNER SNACK OR DESSERT?

Many toddlers look forward to an after-dinner snack. Ideally, this snack should take place at least an hour after dinnertime (e.g., after bath routine). If your toddler likes to have "dessert" after dinner, then serve the dessert as the after-dinner snack. If, however, your toddler struggles with eating her proper food at mealtime, then offer a "more nutritionally complete" dessert for bedtime snack. For example:

- 1 pudding cup with 3–4 vanilla wafers
- 1 cup "warm" chocolate made with milk (hot chocolate, just not too hot), with whipped cream on top
- 1 fruited cereal bar or 2 Fig Newton cookies with milk
- ½ cup low-fat frozen yogurt or ice cream with diced fruit—try adding some sprinkles or sugary cereal such as Fruity Cheerios on top
- Strawberries and whipped cream (or even any fruit cup and whipped cream)
- Oatmeal raisin cookie and milk
- Molasses cookies
- Bowl of cereal and milk

- Banana Fondue: melt peanut butter in a microwave, cut a banana into wheels, and have your toddler dip them in the melted peanut butter with a toothpick.
- Leftover blueberry pancake: sprinkle some powdered sugar on two pancakes, put them together like a sandwich, and cut in half. Delicious! This works well with strawberry jam or maple butter in between as well.

Don't fall into the trap of using dessert as a reward for eating a good dinner. This leaves the toddler to eat her proper food mindlessly, and end up eating too much with the added dessert. Holding out on dessert makes it the "forbidden fruit," which then appears to the toddler as more important than the other food she should be eating. If you have established a good rhythm with your mealtime routine, you will find that on some nights, she will eat more of her main meal and a bit of dessert, and on others it will be the opposite.

APPLYING THE PICK-YOUR-PROTEIN METHOD WITH CONVENIENT FAVORITES

So often parents come into the office asking for quick, healthy convenience foods they can prepare in a hurry for their toddler. Today, we are fortunate to have multiple options available to choose from and keep on hand when we just can't seem to pull together a homemade meal. Check out the list below of well-recognized brand name foods, and plan your toddler meals according to age and amount to serve as we did above using the picking method. Be sure to add on the calcium by offering milk with the meal.

START WITH (PICK YOUR PROTEIN)	ADD
Annie's Whole Wheat Macaroni and Cheese	Broccoli florets, fresh or frozen
Mrs. T's Potato and Cheese Pierogies	Frozen spring peas and carrots
Blake's Chicken Pot Pie (liquid strained if needed)	Motts all natural applesauce with cinnamon
Blake's Organic Shepherd's Pie	Mozzarella cheese stick + slice of Italian bread
Trader Joe's Vegetarian Lentil Soup	Warmed flour tortilla with cheese
Applegate Farms Nitrite-Free hot dogs (cut into quarters)	Bush's Homestyle Baked Beans
Boar's Head honey maple turkey slices, rolled up	Ellio's cheese pizza squares cut in strips
Bell and Evans All Natural Chicken Nuggets	Mashed potatoes + soft-cooked frozen green beans

START WITH (PICK YOUR PROTEIN)	ADD
Progresso Italian Wedding Soup (strained if needed)	Dole diced peaches packed in 100% fruit juice
Wellshire Farms Turkey Maple Sausages (cut in bite size)	Stonyfield Farms Yogurt Squeezers
Mama Leone's Cheese or Beef Ravioli	Peter Rabbit Mango Peach Squeezer
Sabra Classic Hummus	Breton Whole Grain Crackers + sliced pears
Coleman Natural Organic Frozen Meatballs	Wacky Mac Veggie Spirals with parmesan
Shredded rotisserie chicken	1 ear of corn on the cob + mashed potatoes
Jones Turkey Sausage Links	Arnold 100% Whole Wheat Bread, toasted with jelly and butter
Blue Horizon Salmon Cake Bites	Frozen steamed broccoli and cauliflower with vegetable oil
Cracker Barrel Cheese Cuts	Annie's Tomato and Stars plus multigrain crackers
Michael Angelo's All Natural Meat Lasagna	Cauliflower and broccoli, diced together
Annie's Rising Crust Pizza	Sliced grapes and apple wedges (sticks for the one-year-old)

You might be asking yourself, "What makes the foods listed above good choices, and why do they make nutritional sense?" Part of my job is to help families find solutions to the never-ending battle of "what do I feed my child?" I do this by providing name brands of foods I think are decent choices; however, it is also important for parents to understand why they are a good choice. Teaching families how to read a food label, or more importantly, an ingredient list, can be an eye opening experience. It really forces you to take stock of what you are allowing your little toddler to put in her little body.

The convenience food list above is not exhaustive. It is, however, full of good ideas that you can continue to build on, as long as you too learn to read food labels. Here are some points to consider:

The ingredient list. The first thing my eyes dart to when I pick up a product is the length of the ingredient list. In general, the longer the list, the more processed the food. Take a minute to carefully look at the ingredients, as sometimes the list is long because the product simply contains so many things. If you find you can't pronounce half the ingredients listed, then it's probably best to put it back.

Trans-fats? The next thing I look for is trans-fats or hydrogenated fat. Even if the nutrition facts label tells you there are zero grams of trans-fat, I always scroll down to the list of ingredients and see for myself.

Labeling laws allow for a certain amount of trans-fats to be used to make a product before they have to claim the product contains any. A product label can say it has zero trans fats if it contains less than .5 grams per serving. If I see any hydrogenated oils such as partially hydrogenated soybean or cottonseed oil, I put it back.

Where's the fiber? On the nutrition facts label, under carbohydrates, you will see the amount of grams of dietary fiber listed. My eyes then take me back to the ingredient list to see if the fiber is a functional fiber, such as inulin or fructooligosaccharides, or if it is natural—derived from whole-wheat flour, fruits, vegetables, or other whole grains. If the product contains some natural fiber, then it ends up in the cart—if, however, it contains fake fibers that can cause gastrointestinal distress, then it ends up on the shelf.

Have a keen eye. In general, I try to avoid products that contain any of the following ingredients: high-fructose corn syrup, organic brown rice syrup,[3] saccharin, aspartame, titanium dioxide, monosodium glutamate, and soy protein isolates. Note that I said "in general." There are always going to be circumstances

---

3. Recently, we have learned that organic toddler formulas containing organic brown rice syrup had twenty to thirty times more arsenic than other toddler fomulas due to the brown rice syrup. This ingredient is also being used in organic packaged foods, cereal bars, and some gluten-free products that are currently undergoing laboratory testing by scientists. For now, it is best to avoid overconsumption of brown rice syrup in food products until we learn more about it.

when you just can't avoid them, and that is OK. For instance, if your toddler is struggling to gain weight and the food he loves has some soy protein isolates listed in the ingredients, then it's best to allow him to have it. Just try and work on finding a healthier equivalent, or even better, attempt to make it yourself.

WHEN EATING IS LESS THAN PERFECT: VITAMINS, MINERALS, AND SUPPLEMENTS—OH MY!

Every family that comes into my office with a toddler asks if he or she should take a vitamin every day, and if yes, which ones. In general, most toddlers can benefit from a daily multivitamin as their patterns of eating can vary so significantly from day to day. I explain to parents that the vitamin supplements should not be given to replace nutrients from whole foods day to day, but instead should be considered a safety blanket to prevent deficiencies on the days that the food just doesn't seem to add up. It is always important to remember that taking vitamin supplements is not the same as eating the food that provides the vitamins. The food itself often has components to it, such as antioxidants, that are disease-preventing and health-promoting. If your toddler refuses to eat sweet potatoes, don't give up on orange vegetables altogether in favor of a vitamin. Keep trying to offer other good real food sources of vitamin

A, such as carrots, watermelon, mango, or even apricots. Truth be told, the only vitamin most toddlers will *need* to supplement every day is vitamin D, as we discussed in chapter three. As a rule of thumb, I tell parents to find a multivitamin (MVI) that contains 400 IU of vitamin D and up to 100 percent of the recommended daily value for all vitamins to avoid toxicity.

Picking the right vitamin for your toddler

Here are a few things to consider when choosing a multivitamin:

1. Can she chew and swallow it without choking? Some younger toddlers might still need to rely on a liquid multivitamin to take it safely each day. If you are confident your toddler can chew a gummy vitamin, I always tell parents to cut it in half with scissors and allow her to chew one piece at a time. Be sure your toddler is brushing her teeth regularly, as gummy vitamins do contain sugar.

2. Does your toddler skip over meat at most or all of his meals? If yes, then he would need to take a daily multivitamin that includes the minerals zinc and possibly iron. Check with your pediatrician to see if your toddler needs an iron supplement. It is extremely important for parents to know that *none*

of the gummy vitamins available to date contain iron; therefore, you will have to rely on a chewable multivitamin and mineral complex, or your pediatrician will prescribe a liquid iron supplement.

3. Not all vitamins are created equal. In general, most children's multivitamins, unless labeled a "multivitamin and mineral complex," are made up of mostly fat- and water-soluble vitamins. They do not typically have calcium, magnesium, or phosphorus in them. If they do have calcium, it is typically in the amount of 100 mg (only 15 percent of what the toddler needs in a day). As we learned in chapter three, calcium is essential for bone health and often will need to be supplemented separately if your toddler is not meeting her needs from food alone. Talk with a registered dietitian or your pediatrician to be sure your toddler is meeting her calcium needs.

4. If your toddler has been diagnosed with a food allergy or celiac disease and needs to avoid gluten, check the label of your vitamin to be sure it is allergen- and/or gluten-free. Surprisingly, many vitamins contain fish derivatives, so read carefully.

5. Taking a vegetable or fruit powder is not the same as eating the food. Save your money and work on

exposing your toddler to fruits and vegetables each day. Take comfort in knowing that your toddler is most likely meeting his needs of vitamins A and C from fruits alone if he outright refuses his veggies. Always remember, our taste buds change with age—so don't give up on veggies!

6. Don't give your toddler single-ingredient vitamin supplements. For example, avoid using products that provide just one vitamin or mineral, such as vitamin C or zinc. These single vitamin supplements contain very high doses and can provide up to ten times the amount needed for health maintenance. In the case of a toddler, more is never better. The only caveat to this would be if your pediatrician has prescribed iron to your toddler for the treatment of iron deficiency, or in the case of a strict vegan, where vitamin B12 supplements or shots could be needed.

Multivitamins (chewable or gummy): Be sure to check the label to see how many gummies your toddler would need to take in a day for children under four years of age, as each brand varies in amount. For the one-year-old, stick with liquid multivitamins due to the risk of choking. For the two- to three-year-old, watch her closely and cut it in half if necessary.

Multivitamin and complete mineral supplement: Use these vitamins if you feel your toddler skips over most sources of meat, or if your pediatrician has advised you to start giving your toddler a vitamin and mineral supplement.

Calcium: The calcium supplements listed in the table below can be used to provide about 200 mg per day of added calcium, when your toddler is struggling to meet his needs of 700 mg per day. Before relying on a supplement, check out the quick reference list below of calcium content of foods, or refer back to chapter three that covers calcium goals for toddlers. Think of the supplements as a bridge to help meet calcium needs, with the goal being food first.

CALCIUM: COUNT IT UP!

Milk (whole, 2%, 1%, skim, lactose-free)	1 cup: 300 mg
Nonfat dry milk powder	1 teaspoon: 60 mg
Cheese (all slicing varieties)	1 slice: 250–300 mg
Cheese stick (mozzarella, cheddar)	1 stick: 100 mg, 200–250 mg
Cottage cheese	¼ cup: 40 mg
Ricotta	½ cup: 330 mg
Cream cheese	1 tablespoon: 10–15 mg
Ice cream	½ cup: 110 mg
Frozen yogurt	½ cup: 100 mg
Pudding	4-ounce cup: 100–150 mg

Yogurt	4-ounce container: 150 mg
	1 yogurt tube: 100 mg
	8-ounce container: 300 mg
	2.3-ounce Danimal: 100 mg
	1 Dan-o-nino yogurt: 200 mg
	1 YoBaby Whole Milk Drinkable: 400 mg
	1 Earth's Best Organic Fruit Smoothies: 200 mg
Fortified instant oatmeal	1 cup: 350 mg
Tofu processed with calcium salt	½ cup: 200–250 mg
Broccoli	1 cup, cooked: 70 mg
Kale	1 cup, cooked: 95 mg
Pinto beans	1 cup: 100 mg
Fortified cereal	¾ cup: 90–100 mg
Calcium-fortified orange juice	1 cup: 350 mg
Soy milk fortified with calcium	1 cup: 200–300 mg
CLIF Kid ZBar	1 bar: 200 mg
Pizza	1 slice: 100 mg
Macaroni and cheese	1 cup: 95 mg
Cheese ravioli	10 mini-rounds: 60 mg

Vitamin D: For the toddler who is starting to eat a well-balanced diet and is meeting her calcium needs of 700 mg per day with food, consult the following list for good supplements of vitamin D. Remember, if you are relying solely on milk, your toddler would need to drink thirty-two ounces per day to meet her vitamin D needs.

Use the following chart as a guide to selecting a daily supplement. Always check the dose, and be sure the amount you are giving is not more than 100 percent of daily value needs. With most chewable supplements, you will need to give half the dose for a toddler (e.g., half a chewable). Always check the product label as doses can change without warning.

MVI (gummy, chewable, or liquid)	MVI PLUS COMPLETE MINERALS (iron, zinc, phosphorus, magnesium)	CALCIUM AND VITAMIN D	VITAMIN D ONLY
Flintstones Gummies Complete My First Flintstones (take ½ tablet)	Flintstones Complete MVI and Mineral (two- to three-year-olds take ½ tablet)	L'il Critters Calcium chew (200 mg/2)	D-Vi-Sol 400 IU/ml
L'il Critters Gummy Vites	Schiff Children's Multivitamin with Minerals	Rhino Gummy Calci-Bears 200 mg/2 gummies	L'il Critters Vitamin D 800 IU/2 gummies

MVI (gummy, chewable, or liquid)	MVI PLUS COMPLETE MINERALS (iron, zinc, phosphorus, magnesium)	CALCIUM AND VITAMIN D	VITAMIN D ONLY
Up & Up Gummy (Target)	Country Life Liquid Dolphin Pals (no iron)	Up & Up Calcium chews 200 mg/ two gummies	Animal Parade D3 200 IU/ drop
Rainbow Light Just Once Kids Multi-Stars (2 and up); contains 5 mg iron, but no other minerals Rainbow Light Gummy Bear Essentials	Centrum Kids Chewables (take ½ tablet) Rainbow Light NutriStart Multivitamin Powder (½ packet per day)	Rhino Soft Calcium Chews 500 mg/ chew; ideal for toddlers with multiple allergies, limiting intake of all dairy and equivalents	Nature's Made D3 Kids Chewable (400 IU/ chew)

MVI (gummy, chewable, or liquid)	MVI PLUS COMPLETE MINERALS (iron, zinc, phosphorus, magnesium)	CALCIUM AND VITAMIN D	VITAMIN D ONLY
Rhino Gummy Bear Vitamins	Animal Parade GOLD liquid; give only 1 teaspoon per day (not 1 tablespoon)	Animal Parade Calcium Natural Vanilla Sundae 250 mg/2; no vitamin D!	Rainbow Light Sunny Gummies (400 IU/ chew)
Poly-Vi-Sol Poly-Vi-Sol with iron, contains 10 mg iron, but no other minerals		365 Brand Calcium D 200 mg/ two chews	

Now that we have learned to build nutritionally sound meals around the small amounts of food toddlers really need, let's move on to chapter six for more tips on healthy food choices and best bites for toddlers.

A WORD ABOUT FISH OIL SUPPLEMENTS

As we all know, most toddlers unfortunately do not eat fish on a regular basis. Health-food stores and grocery aisles are filled with supplements of fish oil to provide omega-3 fatty acids such as EPA and DHA in place of these fats from food. Unfortunately, not all of these products are regulated by the Food and Drug Administration, and there are no quality standards for doses, nor are there well-defined recommendations of needs in young children. More importantly, despite many of these products claiming to be free of mercury on the label, some contain high quantities of lead, which can be dangerous. As a consumer, there is no way of knowing this, unless you pay to have your supplement tested in a lab. Until we see tighter regulation of these supplements, the jury is out, so keep offering good quality fish at least once per week. If, however, you choose to give your tot a supplement, or you are advised to supplement by a medical professional, be aware that fish oil supplements should be stopped two weeks before any surgery (even dental) or procedure due to concerns with increased risk of bleeding.

CHAPTER SIX

Putting It All Together

Now that we have learned about food introduction, diet expansion, exposure, and the importance of embracing these concepts when feeding a toddler (along with a hefty dose of patience), in addition to how much food really is enough, it's time to consider our options.

What foods are worth the effort, and what quick and easy foods fit into your toddler's busy lifestyle?

THE TOP TEN

By now, you might just be sick of me saying that exposing your toddler to food is one of the most important concepts to embrace during this feeding period; however, I honestly feel it cannot be stressed enough. Research has shown that it can take up to fifteen times for a toddler to be exposed to one food before he is willing to accept it on a daily basis. It is during these times that parents can easily misinterpret a rejection as "I don't like that," when really, their toddler might just be trying to get familiar with that particular food. Staying true to my training as a dietitian, I feel compelled to name the foods I think are worth fifteen exposures (or even more!) because of their nutritional superiority and convenience.

1. Oats

Packed with an excellent dose of soluble fiber to keep your toddler regular, oats are also a good source of protein and iron (when fortified)—and taste delicious when mixed with bone-building calcium. Oatmeal provides satiety, that good old feeling of fullness, which is ideal for our little guys who are hardwired to nibble all day long. The options for oatmeal are endless—instant, quick-cook, steel-cut, or old-fashioned rolled oats. Ideally, for toddlers you want to make the oats soft enough so that minimal chewing is required. Starting with an old-fashioned oat might be better than jumping right to steel-cut. Mixing the oats with a bit of milk while they are cooking on top of the stove will help them soften. Feel free to add a teaspoon of brown sugar, honey, maple syrup, or cinnamon for flavor. Having single packets of fortified instant oatmeal on hand is a great way to make a quick bowl of oatmeal without even reaching for a pot—again, adding a splash of milk while mixing makes for a creamy taste that your toddler will gobble right up.

TOP-RATED CONVENIENT TODDLER BITES

1. Old Fashioned Quaker Oats

2. Quaker Instant Oatmeal

3. Organic 365 Instant Oatmeal, Variety Pack

4. Nature's Path Instant Oatmeal

5. Earth's Best Yummy Tummy Instant Oatmeal, Apple Cinnamon

2. Wild salmon

Health authorities can't say enough when it comes to the importance of including fish in our diets. Buying wild as opposed to farm-raised will help you feel better about some of the toxins that might be found in farm-raised salmon. If you as the parent do not really like fish and find you never have the motivation to prepare salmon (or any other fish for that matter), it is hard to follow the first creed of REAP, role-modeling; therefore, I often suggest to families a few strategies for incorporating fish into their regular diet.

1. Start in the summer. Fish is easy to cook on a grill and won't stink up your house (something my husband immensely appreciates!).

2. Buy some new frozen fish nuggets available on the market and serve with a yummy dipping sauce.

3. Start with a bland, flaky white fish like tilapia or barramundi (U.S.-farmed) before working your way up to more fully flavored fish, like salmon.

4. Pair fish with a familiar fruit flavor (for example, bake or grill fish with fruit salsas)—or for salmon, try something sweet like a teriyaki maple syrup glaze (stir together one tablespoon of teriyaki sauce and one tablespoon of maple syrup).

5. Make it a burger! Look for premade patties at your local grocery store to save you time; pan-sear on top of your stove and then finish off baking in the oven.

TOP-RATED CONVENIENT TODDLER BITES

1. Blue Horizon Salmon Bites (you can start with the pollock and potato minicakes if you feel like easing your toddler into fish a bit more slowly)

2. Henry and Lisa's Salmon Burgers

3. Grocery-store-prepared salmon burgers at the fish counter

4. Happy Bites Salmon Stix

5. Salmon cream cheese spread: mix together one seven-ounce can of salmon and about two to three tablespoons of cream cheese. Season to taste and spread on your toddler's favorite crackers.

6. Mrs. Paul's Healthy Fish Sticks for a white fish alternative

3. Nuts or nut butters

An excellent source of vitamin E, nut butters provide a quick burst of protein, fiber, and magnesium. Nuts are full of monounsaturated fats, which give them an A+ in heart health. When it comes to quantity, a little bit goes a long way, which is perfect for toddlers, notorious for eating small amounts of foods. As a general rule, I advise parents to avoid whole nuts because they are a choking hazard in children. However, adding finely chopped nuts to homemade cookies, breads, or even hot cereals is a great way to expose your toddler to their texture and nutty flavor. The easiest way to offer nuts to a toddler is as a "butter" or spread, e.g., peanut butter. Today there are so many different kinds of nut butters, your toddler is bound to get hooked on one. Beware of hydrogenated oils that are commonly found in spreadable butters. If the label reads "partially hydrogenated oils," skip it and look for one of the brands listed below.

TOP-RATED CONVENIENT TODDLER BITES

1. Skippy's Natural

2. All Natural Peanut Butter & Co. Cinnamon Raisin Swirl

3. Honey Bear All Natural Peanut Butter

4. Blue Diamond Almond Butter

5. 365 Brand Creamy Peanut Butter

6. SunButter Natural Sunflower Butter

7. Justin's Honey Almond Butter

4. Soups

Helping your toddler learn to like soup is a great way to expose her to vegetables, beans, and small pieces of shredded meat. Plus, there are so many versions of pre-made soup that are easy to heat up in a pinch (in place of leftover mac and cheese) on days you might have nothing planned for lunch—or even dinner. Straining the broth will make the soup much easier to eat—so keep your slotted spoon nearby, and be sure it's not too hot before you serve it. Hungry toddlers love to float ice cubes in their soup bowl to help it cool down faster, and be sure to keep some crackers nearby for dipping. My daughter Maggie gets a kick out of fishing for Goldfish in her soup, and now, the Goldfish Colors variety has been remade without any artificial dyes!

TOP-RATED CONVENIENT TODDLER BITES

1. Annie's Certified Organic All Stars (Tomato and Stars)

2. Organic Elmo Vegetable Soup (I add a sprinkle of parmesan cheese to enhance flavor)

3. Progresso Italian Wedding Soup or Chickarina

4. Wolfgang Puck Vegetable Barley

5. Trader Joe's Vegetarian Lentil Soup

6. Annie's Certified Organic Arthur Loops

7. Campbell's Healthy Harvest Tomato Basil

8. Amy's Kitchen Organic Alphabet Soup (be sure to add some grated cheese as this soup only has about eighty calories per serving and it's fat–free, or serve with a wedge of grilled cheese on the side)

5. Eggs

The incredible edible egg is just that. Packed with protein and high in lecithin, an excellent source of gamma-linoleic acid that supports memory and concentration, the egg is a super food that provides staying power (keeps you full) for toddlers who might be prone to beg for food all the time. Try it scrambled, hard-boiled, or even deviled—any way your toddler will accept it. I have been known to make hard-boiled eggs and replace the yolk with a scoop of hummus instead. Better yet, learning to make frittatas (a baked egg dish) is great because you can add all sorts of veggies and flavor to them. Definitely worth a shot for toddlers who love the soft and squishy texture. My colleague Kate Vance has always stood by her recommendation for appetizer quiches (we call them baby quiche). Conveniently prepared and often found in the frozen foods section, just pop them into a toaster oven for a delicious treat at snack time or for a meal.

TOP-RATED CONVENIENT TODDLER BITES

1. 365 Appetizer Quiches

2. Hard-boiled, chopped

3. Scrambled with cheese

4. Mini muffin quiches

5. Deviled with hummus

6. Beans/Legumes

Beans truly are the only food I like to be sneaky about! High in soluble fiber, iron, and complex B vitamins, beans are one of my favorite foods to challenge kids of all ages to learn to like. As we will learn in chapter seven about digestive health, and particularly constipation, beans help keep your toddler regular and can even make harder poops a bit softer. Try them cooked in soups or with pasta, or even blend into bean dip for toddlers who love to dip. My daughter's preschool teacher Miss Sandy brings edamame (soybeans) for lunch every day, and spends time talking to the kids about what they are. Interestingly, when I was walking through the grocery store one day with Maggie, she spotted edamame at the salad bar, and asked to try one. Eagerly, I shuffled over and scooped out a bunch into a take-out bowl, and she readily popped one into her mouth. True to being a toddler, she said she didn't like it, but I was so impressed with how Miss Sandy's role-modeling good eating habits paid off.

TOP-RATED CONVENIENT TODDLER BITES

1. Refried beans spread thinly on a tortilla with melted cheese

2. Amy's Cheese and Bean Nacho Snacks

3. Morning Star Chipotle Black Bean Burger

4. Progresso Macaroni and Bean Soup

5. Trader Joe's Seven Layer Bean Dip

6. Goya Small Red or White Kidney Beans added to favorite soup

7. Zatarain's Reduced Sodium Red Beans and Rice

7. Yogurt

Good yogurt should be a daily staple in the diets of children of all ages. Not just for the calcium, phosphorus, and potassium, but more importantly, for the live active cultures. Live and active cultures in yogurt are essentially the bacteria responsible for turning pasteurized milk into yogurt during the process of fermentation. Tactfully speaking, all yogurts are not created equal; however, any yogurt is better than no yogurt at all. To be sure your toddler is REAPing the benefits of live and active cultures, look for the National Yogurt Association (NYA) seal of approval, which can be found on the yogurt products you buy. Check it out at www.aboutyogurt.com.

Many kids today might not even recognize that yogurt actually comes in a cup—as opposed to a tube, bottle, or crusher. Offer your toddler the purest form of yogurt for as long as you can—and try to avoid the ones with artificial additives (high-fructose corn syrup) and dyes. Food companies today have recognized how many kids have tubes packed in their lunch boxes, and have made some perfectly healthy tubes for tots. Stonyfield

Farms, Horizon, Trader Joe's, and now Yoplait (Simply Yogurt) are perfectly healthy tubes for your tot—with the same ease of packing and fun eating. Even kids can REAP the benefits of high-protein Greek yogurt now, with Chobani Champions being a favorite.

Be sure to offer your twelve- to twenty-month-old full-fat yogurt. Once his diet becomes more varied (which means he is getting enough fat), then it is OK to use both full- and low-fat versions.

TOP-RATED CONVENIENT TODDLER BITES

1. Stonyfield Farms YoKids Squeezers

2. Yoplait Simply Yogurt Tubes

3. Horizon Organic Yogurt Squeezers

4. YoKids and YoBaby Organic Yogurt Cups

5. Wallaby Organic Joey Yogurt Cups

6. Smoothies: YoBaby Whole Milk Drinkables and Stonyfield Farms Probiotic Smoothie

7. All-Natural Brown Cow Cream Top Yogurt

8. YoKids Greek Yogurt

9. Chobani Champions

8. Leafy green vegetables

This might be the hardest food to turn toddlers onto, but well worth the effort. We all know how important eating vegetables like broccoli, spinach, Swiss chard, kale, lettuces, and greens are to our health. But for toddlers, they always seem to be the hardest to like. Personally, I have come to the conclusion that most parents *presume* the toddler won't eat them, so they don't offer them. (I myself am guilty of skipping the spinach as a side dish because I know my kids will eat the broccoli I make instead.) So, I rely on soups, sauces, and baked casseroles to add greens—most of the time, nobody even notices. The truth is that many adults don't even eat these vegetables on a regular basis, so you might have some work to do yourself. And keep in mind not to give up on your toddler while being a good role-model. Just because your toddler doesn't eat these foods today does not mean she will never eat them. As we grow up, our taste buds do too.

TOP-RATED CONVENIENT TODDLER BITES

1. Dr. Praeger's Spinach Pancakes or Broccoli Littles

2. Amy's Organic Vegetable Lasagna

3. Frozen spinach and cheese tortellini or ravioli

4. Blake's Macaroni and Cheese with Vegetables

5. Amy's Broccoli and Cheddar Bake

6. Happy Bites Veggie Tots

7. Garden Lites Roasted Vegetable Souffle

9. Bright orange or yellow fruits and vegetables

A superior source of vitamins A and C, bright yellow and orange vegetables get their famous color from the high content of beta-carotene—and yes, your toddler can turn orange if he eats too much of these! Luckily, the orange hue is mostly contained to the palms of his hands and possibly cheeks. Even better news is that hypercarotenemia goes away and is harmless.

These antioxidant rich foods should be eaten daily, as vitamin A is an essential nutrient for immunity, vision, and cell function. Some of the favorites are carrots, yellow and orange peppers, sweet potatoes, squash (all varieties), mango, cantaloupe, pumpkin, and mixed vegetables. I try to offer a good source twice a day—one at lunch and one for sure with dinner.

I rely heavily on precut melons. Whenever I am at the grocery store, I pick up a few containers to have on hand when my kids come rushing at me for a snack before dinner.

TOP-RATED CONVENIENT TODDLER BITES

1. Dr. Praeger's Sweet Potato Pancakes

2. Alexia Sweet Potato Fries

3. Alexia Sweet Potato Puffs

4. Ian's Sweet Potato Fries

5. Dr. Praeger's Sweet Potato Littles

10. Berries

An excellent source of fiber and readily accepted by most toddlers, berries are truly a super fruit that are portable, require minimal preparation, taste sweet, and are perfectly nutritious. Today, it's easy to rotate through a variety of fresh berries, as grocery stores all over are shipping berries in from warm places. Even better, you always have access to fresh berries in the freezer section that can thaw in no time and be added to breads, muffins, waffles, pancakes, smoothies, or even salads. If your toddler is stuck on fruit snacks, I challenge you to pack a small container of berries in their place with her lunch for preschool or day care, or offer in place of fruit snacks at home. This one small change may lead to less constipation, tummy aches, and definitely less cavities and gum disease.

TOP-RATED CONVENIENT TODDLER BITES (ASIDE FROM THE FRESH FRUIT ITSELF)

1. Earth's Best Organic Fruit Yogurt Smoothies— Mixed Berry (Pouch)

2. Motts Healthy Harvest Blueberry, Mixed Berry, or Summer Strawberry Applesauce

3. Stonyfield Organic Strawberry-licious Frozen Yogurt

4. Van's Organic Blueberry Frozen Waffles

5. Raspberries, strawberries, and whipped cream (chop up strawberries and mix into whipped cream—toddlers love when the whipped cream turns pink!)

6. Berry-flavored cereal bars

7. Nabisco Blueberry Brown Sugar Fruit Thins

A NOTE ON DIET EXPANSION

Some of the top-rated foods mentioned previously might be totally new and intimidating to you when you think of giving them to your tot. For some, you might not even eat these foods yourself on a daily basis! Keep in mind the three concepts we have talked about throughout the book that can help you approach offering new foods. Remember to:

Introduce: Offer food without an agenda and without being invested in what your toddler decides to do once you put the food in front of him. The more you do this, the easier it will become.

Expose: Despite all of your inner voices telling you to abandon ship and just keep serving what she likes—expose your toddler repeatedly to at least one new food a week. Start by committing to one of the foods listed above, and see how it goes. You might be surprised to see how willingly your toddler responds to seeing new foods each week.

Expand: Diet exposure and expansion are never-ending tasks. When people buy a house, they soon realize that the work is never really done. There is "always something" to improve or fix, and the list just keeps getting bigger. The same is true for building a variety of foods into your toddler's diet. Nothing happens overnight! If you can manage to stay consistent with your approach to feeding, particularly after reading this book, you have already won half the battle. Think of diet expansion as a journey—each food you gain along the way is a success.

Getting other family members on board with your plan is crucial to being successful when feeding a toddler. This can go beyond just your spouse if you rely on multiple family members to care for your child in your absence. If there is someone in your toddler's life who cares for her regularly and consistently caters to her when you are not around, that is only going to make it harder for you not to do the same. Sit down with that family member and explain a few important points about what your goals are for your toddler. I completely understand it is a fine line to walk—this person is doing you a huge favor by caring for your child, so it is hard not to feel like a bossy parent. This is especially true for doting grandparents who love to spoil their grandchildren with never-ending snacks and sweets!

The best approach for parents in this situation is to start by asking the caregiver to offer only two choices at mealtimes to avoid the "What would you like for a snack?" question and instead have them say, "Julie, it is snack time; you can have a yogurt or a cheese stick," and remind the person what an impact he or she can have on your toddler simply by sitting at a table to eat together.

Learn to make a few basic meals

While this book offers solid ideas for convenience foods and semi-prepared foods, learning to have at least five recipes in your repertoire to make from scratch is ideal. I always recommend to parents to learn to cook something fresh that their toddler loves but that is often purchased frozen or premade.

First, make a list of the things you buy on a weekly basis that are commercially prepared; then pick one item on that list and learn to make it from scratch. For example, here are some items you may buy on a weekly basis:

Breaded chicken (nugget, finger, cutlet, patty)
Frozen family entrée (e.g., lasagna, beef and macaroni, shepherd's pie)

Frozen meatballs
Boxed macaroni and cheese
Canned soup
Frozen waffles or pancakes

Then, decide which one you will learn to cook yourself for the family.

As we have seen from the lists above, there are many commercially prepared convenience foods that are completely healthy. However, there are many that are not. On average, frozen meatballs might have up to fifteen different ingredients, and frozen waffles might be made with trans-fats such as partially hydrogenated oils—which you won't find in your pantry. Also, making foods from scratch gives you the opportunity to show toddlers what non-processed food tastes like (a big concept often overlooked in this generation). Moreover, the foods you wrote down are most likely to be eaten on a regular basis; therefore, the more natural, the better. Please don't interpret this as me saying you can never use commercially prepared foods in the name of health perfection. However, for foods your toddler regularly accepts and enjoys, buy the least processed brand (with the least additives) or, better yet, cook them from scratch.

Try any of these easy recipes for popular toddler foods listed above.

The Breaded Chicken Cutlet/Nugget

By using organic chicken and a blend of Italian-seasoned and whole-wheat bread crumbs, you can really improve the nutritional quality of "breaded meat" to a top-rated toddler meal. Using olive oil to pan fry is best and completely changes the fat profile of frozen breaded chicken.

These chicken pieces are fun to dip for people of all ages—we always have ketchup on hand, but don't be afraid to try BBQ sauce (we love Stubbs), Worcestershire sauce, or honey mustard in its place. Allow your toddler to squeeze honey into a bowl and add a teaspoon of Dijon mustard and stir!

1 pound organic chicken cutlets or tenderloins, sliced thin
2 eggs, beaten and 1 tablespoon mayonnaise, stirred together
2–3 tablespoons olive oil for pan frying
¾ cup Italian-seasoned bread crumbs plus ¼ cup whole-wheat bread crumbs plus 1 tablespoon parmesan cheese, mixed together in a baking dish

Preheat oven to 350 degrees. Add chicken to the dish of beaten eggs and mayo; soak well to be sure chicken is covered in egg wash. Heat 2 tablespoons olive oil in nonstick sauté pan. Dip the chicken pieces one by one in the mixture of bread crumbs and parmesan cheese. Add each chicken piece to hot pan and cook on each side for 2 to 3 minutes, or until light golden brown. Remove each chicken piece and place on baking sheet. Bake the chicken for 10 to 12 minutes to cook through thoroughly. Slice in small pieces and serve with cooked carrots and/or broccoli and sweet potato fries.

MAKE IT A NEW MEAL

Simply by squeezing sliced lemons over the chicken before you put it in the oven to bake, you are in one swift step exposing your toddler's palate (and therefore expanding his food choices) by making lemon chicken. If you were to go back to the chart you filled out in chapter one, you could add next to "chicken" another variety of the foods he accepts.

EXPAND ON THE NEW FLAVOR/TEXTURE

If your toddler likes the lemon flavor of breaded chicken—after at least ten attempts at trying it!—then try doing the same recipe with a white fish such as cod, sole, or tilapia.

Homemade Macaroni and Cheese

I admit that my kids will always prefer boxed mac and cheese over homemade any day (thanks, Annie!). However, this does not stop me from making the creamier version of from-scratch mac and cheese that I love so much. Making mac and cheese from scratch allows you to switch up the pasta shapes and introduce new flavors of cheeses without anyone protesting about the new flavors. It is much easier to add half a cup of shredded extra sharp cheddar or even smoked gouda to the mix than cutting a slice and offering it alone. (Adapted from Vineyard Seasons, *by Susan Branch.)*

1 (1-pound) box small shells, elbows, or pipettes
2 eggs
½ teaspoon salt
¼ teaspoon cayenne pepper
2 teaspoons dry mustard
2 ½ cups half-and-half
1 ½ pounds of shredded extra sharp cheddar cheese

Preheat oven to 350 degrees. Cook and drain the pasta. In a large mixing bowl, beat the eggs with salt, pepper, and dry mustard. Stir in the half and half and then the grated cheese. Pour cooked pasta into a buttered casserole dish, and then pour cheese and egg mixture over pasta. Bake in oven at 350 degrees for 30 minutes. Before removing from oven, set broiler to high and let top brown slightly for 1 to 2 minutes. Let cool before serving with sliced cucumbers or green beans.

MAKE IT A NEW MEAL

Simply by adding one cup of cooked, chopped broccoli florets and even some cooked diced chicken, you have turned basic mac and cheese into a casserole loaded with vitamin C and protein.

EXPAND ON THE NEW FLAVOR/TEXTURE

If your toddler accepts the mixed consistency of pasta, veggies, and chicken, try making another casserole with different shaped pasta and a new vegetable such as peas.

Homemade Meatballs

Meatballs are a favored food of toddlers because of their squishy consistency and are a very easy way to get in a day's worth of protein, as well as a hefty dose of iron and zinc if you choose beef.

Making your own meatballs minimizes your toddler's exposure to many filler proteins used by food manufacturing companies (e.g., hydrolyzed soy protein), in addition to allowing you to create the perfect size ball: the small ball is always preferred in our house. On busy weeknights when I just can't seem to get it together for a real sit-down dinner, I pull out some homemade meatballs and stick them on toothpicks (not appropriate for the one-year-old and with supervision for the two-year-old), and serve with a side of tomato sauce for dipping. My kids love this with fresh baby carrots sticks (thin sliced), sliced cucumbers, and a stick of mozzarella cheese.

1 pound 85% lean grass-fed beef (if available)
2 eggs, cracked
¼ cup Pecorino Romano finely grated cheese
    (OK to use parmesan in place)
1 slice white sandwich bread (no crusts) or roll
    (e.g., hot dog), pulled apart and soaked in 2
    tablespoons milk
⅛–¼ cup Italian-seasoned bread crumbs
1 teaspoon salt
1 teaspoon oregano
2 teaspoons black pepper
2 teaspoons garlic powder

1–2 tablespoons olive oil for cooking
Dorot frozen parsley and garlic cubes

Preheat oven to 325 degrees (convection bake if available). Add all ingredients except oil and parsley and garlic cubes to a large mixing bowl and mix together with your hands. The mixture should be semi "wet," but you should still be able to roll small meatballs. Heat oil in large nonstick sauté pan over medium-high heat. Add 1 to 2 frozen garlic and parsley cubes to oil, and let dissolve (takes a minute). Add meatballs to sauté pan (working in batches if necessary), and brown on all sides, cooking for 5 to 7 minutes. Transfer meatballs with a slotted spoon to baking sheet, and place in oven to finish cooking for about 15 minutes. Place in favorite tomato sauce on top of stove or freeze for future use.

MAKE IT A NEW MEAL

Simply switch out the ground beef for ground chicken or turkey and add some finely chopped fresh parsley and baby spinach to the mixture for a wonderful flavor.

EXPAND ON THE NEW FLAVOR/TEXTURE

Meatloaf is essentially the same thing as one giant meatball cut in loaf-size pieces, and of course, served without pasta. If your toddler enjoys the squishy consistency of meatballs with a tomato sauce flavor, try making meatloaf and serving it in small, cut-up pieces with a side of mashed potatoes in place of pasta.

Patsy's Chicken Meatballs

1 pound ground chicken (not fat-free or extra lean)
1 egg
¼ cup bread crumbs, Italian-seasoned
1 slice bread, softened with milk
2 tablespoons chopped fresh flat-leaf
   Italian parsley
4 cloves garlic, mashed with a heavy knife, and
   chopped fine
2 tablespoons grated parmesan cheese
¼ teaspoon salt
¼ teaspoon pepper
1 yellow onion, chopped
Olive oil for frying

Combine all ingredients except onion and olive oil in bowl. Mix thoroughly; mixture will feel quite sticky because the chicken consistency is soft; a wooden spoon helps the mixture. Using warm running water to coat your hands, form the mixture into small meatballs and place all on a microwaveable plate. Microwave meatballs about 4 minutes; check—some may need turning—and microwave 1 more minute. In a browning skillet, sauté onion in olive oil. Add meatballs to skillet and carefully get a good brown to the outside of the meatballs. Add onions and meatballs to tomato sauce; cook on low heat for 30 minutes.

Chicken Noodle Soup

There is nothing better than coming home to the smell of homemade soup. My mother Patsy is the queen of all soups and is truly my inspiration in the kitchen. Despite all the cookbooks she has purchased or handed down over the years, I still choose to pick up the phone and ask her a soup question in person (back in high school I was guilty of even having her paged at the grocery store to ask a burning question about soup for dinner!). Also a dish that can be made ahead of time and popped right out of the fridge onto the stove, soup could be the best meal you learn how to make for a number of reasons: high nutritional value, ease of including veggies, and simplicity in serving. Once you learn the basics of making one soup, you can pretty much make any kind of soup you like. Have some garlic bread on hand or buy fresh bread from a local bakery, and you have a meal in minutes. Learn to make creamier soups that might be laden with excess fat and calories with potato puree, sharp grated cheese, and 2 percent milk. Toddlers love homemade potato soup because of its thick consistency and scrumptious flavor.

2 chicken breasts, split, boned, skinless
1 bunch celery, finely chopped (save leaves/stems)
3 Dorot frozen parsley cubes
2–3 Dorot frozen garlic cubes
1–2 teaspoons kosher salt
1 large yellow onion, peeled and finely chopped
Cooking oil
3–4 carrots, peeled and chopped into small pieces
1 cup fresh spinach or Swiss chard, finely chopped
2 (14.5-ounce) cans store-bought chicken broth
1 box ditalini or acini di pepe soup noodles

Put raw chicken breasts into a pot with water to cover them completely. Add celery leaves, parsley and garlic cubes, and kosher salt. Bring to a boil on high heat, uncovered. Turn to medium heat and allow water to be at a rolling boil for about 15 minutes. In the meantime, add cooking oil to soup pot on medium heat and sauté finely chopped onion until translucent. Add carrots and celery and stir around to allow them to soften and simmer. Add a splash of canned chicken stock to prevent them from sticking to bottom of pot. Add chopped spinach or Swiss chard. Turn boiling chicken breasts to low simmer and cover. Continue to cook for about 30 minutes. Remove chicken breasts from pot of boiling water and place in a large bowl. Return pot of "stock" to a boil for about another 45 minutes. Shred chicken with a fork into small pieces and add to carrot, celery, and onion mixture. Pour 1 can of store-bought chicken broth into pot of chicken and veggies. Simmer on low for about 20 minutes. In a separate pot, boil water for small pasta noodles. Cook and drain as directed on package. Spoon homemade chicken stock by the ladle into soup mixture for desired consistency. Add cooked pasta in the final step. Serve with warm bread and butter or a sprinkle of parmesan cheese.

MAKE IT A NEW MEAL

Simply by replacing the pasta with either cooked white or brown rice you are making a new meal of chicken rice soup, yet again exposing your toddler to another variety of chicken soup and expanding his diet.

EXPAND ON THE NEW FLAVOR/TEXTURE

Use the base recipe above with rice and add only half a can of store-bought chicken broth/stock (about 7 ounces) and replace the other half with one, 14.5-ounce can of diced tomatoes. Add 1 can of corn, drained, and ½ can of Goya petite red kidney beans for a quick rendition of tortilla soup. Instead of bread, serve multigrain tortilla chips for dipping and sprinkle grated cheddar cheese on top.

Homemade Pancakes

Do you ever wonder why the pancakes you eat at a diner are always better than the boxed mix you have in your house? They all seem to have this spongy texture that store box mixes always yield as fluffy. Making pancakes from scratch allows you to replicate this texture and gives your toddler a break from the frozen varieties that tend to be made with hydrogenated oils and even some processed sugars.

1 ½ cups all-purpose flour + 1 tablespoon wheat
   germ (optional)
½ teaspoon salt
1 tablespoon + 1 teaspoon baking powder
1 tablespoon sugar
1 egg, lightly beaten

1 ½ cups milk

3 tablespoons + 1 teaspoon melted butter

In a large mixing bowl, add flour, salt, baking powder, and sugar. Shake together. Add beaten egg, milk, and 3 tablespoons melted butter. Stir together gently (avoid over-stirring). Heat 1 teaspoon butter, PAM, or canola oil over medium heat on a nonstick skillet or griddle. Using a soup ladle, scoop pancake batter onto hot griddle or skillet, and flip when you see bubbles appear. Cook until light brown. Serve immediately with a side of banana wheels, fresh berries, or even a shake of cinnamon and powdered sugar.

MAKE IT A NEW MEAL

For a seasonal twist, try adding some fresh blueberries to the mix or even some grated apples. By accepting different kinds of pancakes, you are expanding your toddler's diet with yet another option for early-morning mealtime.

EXPAND ON THE NEW FLAVOR/TEXTURE

If you find your toddler is loving pancakes in the morning, take it a step further and try making crepes instead. The best thing about crepes is that they can be filled with all sorts of yummy fillings, such as Nutella, peanut butter and bananas, strawberry jam, or even ricotta cheese mixed with cinnamon sugar or honey.

THIRTY PANTRY-READY SURVIVAL MEALS

While you are learning to prepare some meals from scratch and expose your toddler to what real, proper food tastes like, take a look below at these pantry-ready survival meals for toddlers—to be applied morning, noon, or night!

It's 4:40, you just get home, drop your bag in the front hallway, and realize—it's dinnertime. Looking at your tired toddler, you quickly come to the conclusion that your perfectly planned dinner of baked chicken, rice, and broccoli will just not work for tonight, despite the potential for it to be ready in under thirty minutes (shout out to Rachel!).

You realize that if you give her snack-type food now, she probably won't eat much of the nutritionally balanced dinner you planned on making, which will inevitably grate on your very last nerve. So you instinctively switch gears and decide to throw together a quick, healthy "meal" in under ten minutes and save the snack for later.

Below is a list of pantry-ready survival meals for toddlers that can be served morning, noon, or night, when you're in a pinch for something fast that is healthy and, well, resembles a toddler-sized meal.

- Be sure to offer a half cup of whole milk with each of these meals to help your tot meet his daily needs for calcium. For the non-milk drinkers, refer to chapter five's complete list of good sources of calcium to add to these meals in place of milk.
- Remember to offer whole grains most of the time for crackers, cereals, breads, and rice to maximize micronutrient content.
- The amount of foods listed here is a place to start. Offer your toddler more if she is still hungry.
- If you do use these meals frequently, well-balanced snacks need to be provided three times per day in order for your toddler to meet his daily calorie requirements. Refer back to chapter five for healthy toddler snacks.

Looking at the list below, it is easy to see that these are not "home-cooked," five-star meals. The meals do, however, contain real food, which is always going to be more nutritionally complete and taste better than fast food or prepackaged toddler meals. As we know, fresh foods can have a tremendous impact on overall health and immunity. In chapter seven, we will learn that a high-quality diet that includes fresh fruits, vegetables, whole grains, and healthy fats will have an even bigger impact on your toddler's overall digestive health.

- 1–2 slice(s) deli ham, rolled up
- 4-ounce container rice pudding (Kozy Shack)
- 2 tablespoons golden raisins (for the toddler under two, substitute 1 sliced banana)

- 2 tablespoons canned white meat chicken mixed with mayonnaise (or plain)
- ½ whole-wheat English muffin with butter
- 4 ounces Dole diced pineapple

- 2 small prepared meatballs, with a side of tomato sauce to dip (or grape jelly)
- 1 slice of garlic bread with cheese
- 1 tablespoon avocado cubes

- 2 tablespoons tuna fish mixed with ranch dressing
- Sliced cucumbers or pickles
- 4–5 whole-grain crackers

- 1 egg, hard-boiled and chopped
- ½ cinnamon toaster waffle with butter
- 5 cantaloupe cubes cut in small pieces

- 2 tablespoons chopped rotisserie chicken
- 3 tablespoons frozen mixed vegetables with butter
- 8–10 grapes cut in half or quarters to prevent choking

- 1 cheddar cheese stick, sliced lengthwise
- ¼ cup strained soup on hand
- ½ apple, sliced into sticks
- 1 handful of veggie sticks

- ½ turkey or all-beef nitrate-free hot dog, sliced down the middle and quartered
- ½ sweet potato, mashed with butter and cinnamon
- ½ soft fresh pear, sliced in small cubes or 1 container diced pears

- ½ cup ricotta cheese with cinnamon and honey or agave
- 2 tablespoons berries
- ¼ cup dried cereal

- 1 small tortilla
- 1 tablespoon refried beans spread thin +1 handful shredded cheddar cheese, warmed
- 4-ounce container mandarin oranges

- 2–3 premade mini quiches (with your toddler's favorite flavors)
- 2–3 tablespoons blueberries
- ½ slice whole wheat bread with butter

- 3 tablespoons macaroni and cheese
- 2–3 tablespoons cooked broccoli
- 1 Motts Healthy Harvest Peach Medley Applesauce

- 3 Bagel Bites (add a pinch of your toddler's favorite cheese before cooking)
- 2 tablespoons green peas
- 2 tablespoons diced mango

- 4 tablespoons cooked orzo + ½ cup store-bought chicken broth, warmed
- 2 tablespoons chopped fresh spinach (or whatever frozen vegetable you have in the house), added to soup
- ¼–½ soft pita bread (Arnold Pita Thins are yummy)

- ½ grilled cheese sandwich with 1 slice honey maple turkey
- 4–5 Tater Tots
- 4–5 cubes watermelon, cut into small pieces

- 2 tablespoons hummus plus 3 pieces Hormel All Natural Pepperoni
- 5–7 Wheat Thins
- 2–3 tablespoons diced strawberries

- 4–5 tablespoons lentil soup (or "best bet" canned soup in pantry)
- 1 roll with butter
- Diced peaches

- 1 baked potato, with shredded cheese and butter
- Leftover protein, such as chicken, diced
- 2 tablespoons green beans with butter

- 1 scrambled egg with cheese
- ½ mini bagel with cream cheese
- 1 cubed kiwi

Cheesy rice: mix 3 tablespoons cooked brown minute
   rice (or leftover rice) plus shredded cheese
1 turkey breakfast sausage
5 cubes honeydew melon, chopped

1 slice pumpkin or banana bread with cream cheese
   or butter
2 tablespoons craisins or raspberries
1 slice deli turkey or chicken

Boar's Head all-beef hot dog, sliced lengthwise and
   cut in half
Ketchup to dip
2–3 tablespoons baked beans
Petite diced cooked carrots with butter

1 tablespoon peanut butter (spread thin) +
   strawberry jam
1 slice soft whole-grain bread
½ banana + 6 fresh cherries, pitted and diced

- 2 Happy Bites Salmon Sticks
- 10–15 oven-baked French fries
- Mixed fruit cup

- 5 mini cheese ravioli with tomato sauce for dipping
- ¼ cup steamed zucchini with olive oil and parmesan cheese
- 8–10 black olives (cut in half or presliced)

- 3 pork and vegetable pot stickers (frozen)
- 4 tablespoons brown rice
- 2 tablespoons diced pineapple + 2 tablespoons green peas

- 3 potato and cheese pierogies
- 4 ounces applesauce
- 3 tablespoons steamed broccoli

- 1 English muffin half, with tomato sauce and cheese (toasted)
- 3 tablespoons blueberries
- 1 handful puffed corn/rice (Pirate's Booty)

- 2 turkey meatballs (frozen)
- ¼ cup penne pasta, cooked
- 2 tablespoons jarred (or homemade) tomato or Alfredo sauce
- 2–3 tablespoons finely chopped fresh spinach, added to sauce

- 2 Freebird Chicken Tenders, BBQ dipping sauce
- 6 honey wheat pretzels
- 3 tablespoons chopped strawberries + 3 honeydew melon cubes

CHAPTER SEVEN

Your Toddler's Digestive Health

One of the biggest milestones three-year-olds will cross in their lifetimes is learning to use a potty. Parents often have anxieties surrounding their toddler's ability to potty train and worry if they will be able to actually "do it." Many toddlers will be potty-trained by three and a half, and others might take a bit longer. No matter how long it takes your child, supporting their digestive health is of the utmost importance for successful potty training.

What do I mean when I say digestive health? Your toddler's digestive system (the organs responsible for breaking food down into nutrients that can be absorbed and hence lead to total body growth) depends on a variety of complex nutrients to work properly. More importantly, the kind of food your toddler eats has an impact on the balance of bacteria in the digestive tract. Ideally, bacteria need to be kept in good balance. Better balance means feeling better all around. Most importantly, all foods that go into your toddler's little body can have an impact on how poop is formed. There are foods your toddler can include in her diet each day that can actually make pooping easier (think less straining, softer stool). We will talk about these foods here.

GREAT EXPECTATIONS: THE CHANGE FROM INFANT POOP TO TODDLER POOP

When your toddler was an infant, especially if your infant was breast-fed for a period of time, you probably adjusted into a nice schedule of feeding and changing diapers and could even proudly report how many poops a day your baby had. Infants who were breast-fed might have been pooping bright yellow seedy poops four to six times per day—some pooping even after every feed. I'll never forget the time when my husband Brian came to meet my son Jake and me at my office after work. I had picked him up from day care early, and I was nursing him while working at my desk. When Brian came in, he went right over and picked Jake up, happy to see him after a long day at the office. Within five minutes of being held, Jake exploded all out of his diaper and all over my husband's pink shirt! This was the first time it happened to us, and everyone who was there just laughed knowingly—as if it were no surprise to them at all. Infant pooping was easy, and it happened often. Toddlers, however, are a whole different animal.

See, the diet from infancy to toddlerhood changes from mostly liquids to one that primarily includes table foods, and that change has a tremendous impact on how your toddler poops: both in frequency and consistency. The digestive system now has to actually work at breaking down solid foods into nutrients that can be absorbed. Think of digestion as a washing machine on a super-clean cycle, trying to free your favorite jeans from dried mud or yogurt (blast those yogurt tubes!): churning, mixing, squirting, and then at last spinning out perfectly clean jeans, free from dirt particles. In this analogy, the dirt would be the nutrients absorbed to promote growth (where *does* all the dirt go in a washing machine anyway?), and the jeans would be the product of the process (e.g., the poop).

Once your toddler begins eating more solid food in his diet, you need to lower your expectations on how often he *should* be pooping. And, if we could devise an equation to predict the number of poops a healthy toddler would have in a day, it would look something like this:

Picky toddler = small amounts of food and liquid in = small amounts of poop out

The days of counting poops past two per day are long gone, and some toddlers may go as infrequently as once every three to four days. Take a look at other ways table food changes how your toddler poops:

Color: Poops can and will range in color from light green to mustard yellow to dark brown. You only need to worry about the color of poop if it is whitish, pale gray (think clay), dark black, or you see bright red blood in the toilet.

Odor: The sweet smell of the breast-fed baby's poop is quickly replaced by adult-poop smell once the diet becomes more complex. This is the result of digested food and gas-producing bacteria that are naturally found in your digestive system.

Consistency: Poops can range from soft (like soft-serve ice cream) to formed (like peanut butter or Silly Putty) to hard (like pebbles) in a toddler and can vary from week to week or even day to day. What your toddler eats and drinks and how much she drinks will influence the consistency of her stool. Too little to drink and too little fiber will lead to a harder poop, and too much fluid, especially in the form of sugary fruit juice (as in Marisol's story in chapter four), can lead to diarrhea.

Food particles: Poop is a by-product of what we eat as well as digestive secretions. If certain foods are not completely digested, then parts might show up in your toddler's poop (think corn, watermelon). This is normal and nothing to worry about.

Now that we have talked about digestive changes in toddlerhood, let's take an in-depth look at two of the most common problems seen in toddlers—constipation and diarrhea—and look at how food choices can have a profound influence on both.

CONSTIPATION

The number-one referral pediatricians make to a gastrointestinal (GI) specialist is for constipation. Approximately 25 percent of visits to a pediatric gastroenterologist are due to problems caused by constipation. By definition, constipation is a condition where poops happen infrequently, or formed poop is dry, hard, and often painful to pass. In addition to lack of fluid and dietary fiber, constipation in toddlers can develop from behavioral issues such as stress surrounding potty training, stubbornness to transition from playing to pooping (or even practicing sitting on a potty), to even just simple fear of using the potty. Constipation can also begin after travel or even a viral illness. These are all very real issues that you need to talk to your pediatrician about, with the goal of establishing a consistent routine surrounding potty training.

For the time being, take a few minutes to consider how much fiber your toddler eats each day by answering these few simple questions:

- Does he eat fruits and vegetables on a daily basis?
- Do you buy whole-grain breads regularly?
- Does the cereal he eats have at least two to three grams of fiber per serving?

If you feel like you could not answer yes to each of these questions, then read on to learn about the foods that can make pooping a bit easier.

Fiber: Not just what grandma called roughage

Dietary fiber is the most influential nutrient on the regulation of your toddler's bowel movements. There are two kinds of fiber we can obtain from what we eat: soluble and insoluble fiber. Soluble fiber (think oatmeal, beans) will soak up water and form a gel in your toddler's stomach, making her feel fuller longer, and will even help keep blood sugar in check (which can help mood!). Insoluble fiber (think fruits and whole-wheat bread) will create bulk and help move food along the digestive tract. Fiber is found mostly in legumes, fruits, and vegetables, and naturally in whole-grain oats, cereals, brown rice, and breads. Ideally, toddlers will benefit from a mixture of fiber from both sources on a regular basis.

It cannot be stressed enough that fiber from food will always work better than fiber from supplements. The hard part with feeding almost all toddlers, as you know now, is that their diet can drastically vary from day to day, so some parents might rely on fiber supplements to keep their toddler regular. If you have found that fiber supplements are not working for your toddler, refer to the table on page 233 for some ideas to try in place of supplements.

BEWARE OF INULIN

As the number of functional foods has remarkably increased over the past ten years, you will find many products with added inulin. Inulin is a type of fiber classified as a fructan that comes from chicory root. Inulin can cause serious gas, cramping, and bloating. Be sure to read food labels that tout that fiber has been added for health benefits: if you see inulin on the label, skip it and head for some organic apples instead.

Can my toddler eat too much fiber?

Yes! Toddlers can be a victim of too much fiber. More is not necessarily better. Excess fiber intake in a tiny belly can actually lead to gas, belly aches, and very large stools that are painful to pass. I always caution parents about going overboard, which can happen when you make a big switch to everything whole-grain or all whole-wheat, especially all at once. For example, choosing 100 percent whole-grain bread for sandwiches and toast is necessary, while only using whole-wheat pasta is not. Ideally, you should shoot for giving your toddler half to three-quarters of his grains as whole grains, and the rest can be made up with a mixed variety. In addition, I will always warn parents about getting caught in the high-fiber candy bar aisle (think Fiber One Bars and Kudos Bars). As a rule of thumb, try to have your toddler obtain most of her fiber from whole, natural foods—not processed, engineered foods with a ton of added fiber. Striking the right balance between soluble and insoluble fibers from foods is the key to your toddler's digestive health.

So how many grams of fiber does your toddler need to eat in a day?

The new fiber DRI for toddlers age one to three years old is 19 grams per day. In our practice, we don't consistently use this reference, as many professionals agree it seems just too high when you take into account how little food toddlers eat in a day. In general, we advise parents to have their toddler eat a minimum of 10 grams of fiber per day. If you find your toddler tolerates more fiber than this over time, then go with it. Just be sure he is drinking enough fluids to move the bulk through his system.

Lastly, when increasing fiber in your toddler's diet, you must be sure he is taking in an adequate amount of fluid. As we have already discussed, thirty-two ounces per day of fluid is plenty, and be sure to include about four to eight ounces as water.

LIKABLE SOURCES OF
FIBER FOR TODDLERS

FOOD	FIBER
CLIF Kid ZBars	3 g/bar
Nutri-Grain Cereal Bars	3 g/bar
Kashi Chocolate Chip Banana Bar	3 g/bar
15 blueberries	2 g
1 tablespoon peanut butter	1 g
1 Eggo Nutri-Grain Honey Oat Waffle	1.5 g
½ cup barley, cooked	3 g
½ cup Trader Joe's vegetarian lentil soup	2.5 g
2 Whole Wheat Fig Newtons	4 g
Applesauce Squeezers	1 g
4–5 peeled apple slices	2 g
1 small banana	2 g
½ medium avocado	4 g
15 raspberries	4 g
½ cup cooked broccoli	2 g
½ cup cooked carrots	3 g
½ cup green peas	4 g
½ cup mashed potatoes	2 g
½ cup pumpkin puree	4 g
½ sweet potato	3 g

FOOD	FIBER
½ cup beans: garbanzo, lima, baked, red kidney, black, pinto, refried	5–7 g
½ kiwi	2 g
½ cup Annie's Whole Grain Mac and Cheese	2.5 g
16 Wheat Thins	3 g
5 slices pear	2 g
2 oatmeal cookies	3 g
2 tablespoons raisins	1 g
¼ cup Sunsweet Plum Amazins	3 g
Breads	
Arnold 100% Whole Wheat	3 g/slice
Freihofer's Stone Ground 100% Whole Wheat	2 g/slice
Arnold Soft Del pita	5 g/pita
Wonder Stoneground 100% Whole Wheat	2 g/slice
Nature's Own Whole Wheat Bread	2 g/slice
Mission Soft Taco Whole Wheat tortillas	3 g /tortilla
Cereals	
Cheerios	3 g per ¾ cup
Multigrain Cheerios	3 g per ¾ cup

FOOD	FIBER
Oatmeal, old-fashioned rolled oats	4 g per ½ cup
Cascadian Farms Cinnamon Crunch	3 g per 1 cup
Quaker Instant Oatmeal	3 g per 1 packet

HOW IT ALL ADDS UP
Shirley's Story

Shirley was three years old and came to our office for instruction on a high-fiber diet. Her family doctor had referred her to see one of the nurse practitioners for constipation. Shirley's mother was struggling with potty training, and Shirley often complained of tummy aches that seemed to be timed with when she had to poop. Mom was wary of starting a daily prescribed laxative, and wanted to learn about how she could make changes to Shirley's diet first, before committing to medicine every day. We got down to business and started to go over what foods she liked and included in her diet each day:

Breakfast	1 waffle with butter and syrup Apple juice
Snack	2 graham crackers with milk

Lunch	SpaghettiOs with hot dogs Diced peaches or apple sauce Apple juice 2 butter cookies
Snack	Raisins or tortilla chips
Dinner	Chicken thigh or leg Mashed potatoes and green beans Milk to drink

Shirley's mom explained that she ate a decent amount of food at each meal but didn't really like to try new things. I asked her if she had explored a different variety of fresh fruits and whole-grain breads, and Mom confessed she had not. We decided to make some small changes to her diet based on the kind of food she already accepted and cut back on the apple juice overall, replacing it with four ounces of pear juice and then water.

Take a look at the chart below that compares Shirley's current diet with the new and improved "higher" fiber diet I recommended:

BEFORE (GRAMS OF FIBER)	AFTER (GRAMS OF FIBER)

Waffle with butter and
  syrup (0 g)
Apple juice (0 g)
	Eggo Nutri-Grain Waffles,
	  Honey Oat (1.5 g)
	6 fresh apple slices (2 g)
	Milk to drink

BEFORE (GRAMS OF FIBER)	AFTER (GRAMS OF FIBER)
2 graham crackers (1 g) Milk	No changes made; familiar foods maintained. Try and alternate milk with yogurt to reap the benefits of live active cultures naturally found in yogurt.
SpaghettiOs with hot dogs (0 g) Diced peaches or apple sauce (1 g) Apple juice 2 butter cookies (0 g)	Annie's P'ghetti Loops with soy meatballs (2 g) ½ diced fresh mango (2 g) 4 ounces pear juice 2 100% Whole Grain Fig Newtons (2 g)
Raisins (1 g) or tortilla chips (0 g)	Kept raisins (1 g), agreed to try multigrain tortilla chips (2 g)
Chicken thigh or leg ¼ cup mashed potatoes (1 g) Green beans (2 g)	Chicken thigh or leg Mashed sweet potato (3 g) Agreed to alternate with peas and carrots mix (3 g)
Fiber Total: 6 g/day	**Fiber Total:** 18.5 g/day

In just a thirty-minute conversation, we were able to come up with a plan that tripled Shirley's fiber intake, without doing a complete overhaul of what she was currently eating! Mom called about five weeks later to report that she liked the mango and multigrain tortilla chips dipped in guacamole—another excellent source of fiber. Shirley did not fall in love with the substitute for SpaghettiOs, so Mom still gave her the brand she liked— just not every day. Instead she tried some homemade tomato soup with soft cooked veggies and ring-shaped noodles, which Shirley was learning to enjoy—she even started to dip some whole wheat crackers in the soup for an extra kick of fiber.

Shirley's mom found that drinking water in place of apple juice helped too, as well as the pear juice. Her poops were softer and she complained of fewer stom-achaches. Occasionally, Shirley would go for several days without a poop, but it was happening much less frequently. In the morning, Shirley's mom started eating her own bowl of oatmeal mixed with a little flaxseed oil and shredded apple. She was so excited when Shirley asked to taste it and exclaimed she liked it! Hopefully that dish will someday be included in her weekly break-fast choices soon.

WHAT ELSE CAN I TRY?

If a high-fiber diet just has not seemed to help your toddler become more regular, try one of the following natural remedies in addition to keeping up with fiber intake for constipation.

Pear juice daily: I know that I have already said that fruit juice should be limited to no more than four to six ounces per day; however, if your toddler is struggling with constipation, then using baby pear juice in the amount of two to four ounces per day is a safe and effective way to help combat constipation. Pear juice, like prune juice, is high in sorbitol, which is a natural laxative that can help promote regularity in your toddler. Be sure to buy pear juice and not nectar, as the juice will have a higher sorbitol content. You will find Gerber pear juice in the baby-food aisle at your supermarket.

Use flaxseed oil when adding fats to food: Flaxseed oil is a lubricant and can help move poop downstream effectively. It is also a decent source of essential fatty acids, so you are getting bang for your buck. Flaxseed oil has to be refrigerated—look for it in the grocery store usually in a refrigerated case at the end of an aisle. Use up to one tablespoon per day added to foods.

Oat bran: I highly recommend including oatmeal in your toddler's diet, but if you can try a quarter cup of cooked oat bran three to four times per week served warm with cinnamon and brown sugar, you might see a difference in how frequently your toddler poops. Look for Mother's Oat Bran, which has a perfect blend of soluble and insoluble fiber with a total of 6 grams of fiber per half cup serving.

Yogurt: Good yogurt is the perfect food to promote digestive health as it naturally contains live active cultures that help regulate digestion. Health care professionals often recommend what is called a "probiotic" supplement that you can purchase at a drug store in powder form. Yogurt, however, naturally contains these probiotics, which essentially are health-promoting bacteria. Recent data has shown us that eating yogurt itself might be better for gut health than simply taking a probiotic powder or capsule alone. Look for probiotic smoothies, and yogurts that do not have a long list of artificial additives and high-fructose corn syrup. Make yogurt a part of each day, and your toddler will be sure to reap its benefits over time.

Add soy milk: If your toddler is a big milk drinker (more than three cups per day), try alternating cow's milk with enriched soy milk. I usually recommend adding one cup of soy milk in place of one cup of cow's milk and going from there. I don't recommend switching entirely to soy milk, as a wide variety of foods in the diet is preferred. Dairy foods such as milk, cheese, and yogurt alone are not constipating, but large amounts of cow's milk in absence of a variety of fruits, vegetables, and whole grains could be contributing to constipation. And soy milk is made from soybeans; therefore, it naturally contains more fiber than milk.

Exercise: Even toddlers need activity. Today, many parents find themselves shuffling their toddler from one place to the next—from day care or preschool to grocery store to home, without ever finding time to let their toddler run around and play. Lack of exercise is one of the most frequently overlooked contributors to constipation. So the next time you pull into the grocery store with your toddler in tow, park far away, hold her hand, and have her walk along side of you if she can. Better yet, when you get home, get outside and play tag!

Get out your grinder: Clean out the coffee beans and finely pulse walnuts, almonds, or macadamia nuts to make a paste and add to cookie, pancake, sweet bread, or waffle mixes. Nuts have natural oils that have a lubricating effect on the GI tract, and add wonderful flavor to foods most toddlers willingly accept.

Cook with garlic and onions: Garlic has a high content of allicin, which helps keep the immune system functioning properly and maintains the integrity of the GI tract. Onion, in the same family as garlic, contains a flavonoid called quercetin that also can contribute to digestive health and overall immunity. Plus, your toddler will appreciate foods that are amplified to taste so delicious.

Stick to a schedule of planned meals and snacks: One thing I repeatedly find when talking with parents of toddlers who are constipated is that they fall into the category of grazers—tots who nibble all day long without ever really eating a "sit-down" meal. As mentioned earlier in the book, toddlers who graze simply don't consume enough calories in the day, and mostly choose snack-type foods that are low in fiber. Also, these grazers tend to compensate for their hunger by drinking more milk—which doesn't always help if they have a limited diet of proper food.

Try Benefiber: Although we always want fiber to come directly from whole foods and not supplements, there are circumstances where some toddlers need a little extra boost. Benefiber is a powdered form of wheat dextrin, a soluble fiber, that does not contain a super-high dose for little bodies. Stir two teaspoons into six ounces of a mixture of apple cider and water, or you can try sprinkling onto foods.

WILL GOING GLUTEN-FREE IMPROVE MY TODDLER'S DIGESTIVE HEALTH?

One trend I see more of when it comes to constipation is the elimination of gluten from the diet. Gluten is the main protein found in wheat, barley, rye, and oats and is well known to cause trouble for children with celiac disease. In celiac disease, the part of the small intestine that is responsible for absorbing nutrients becomes flattened or damaged, leaving the afflicted child undernourished and subsequently with overall poor growth. Other symptoms might include anemia, diarrhea or constipation, fatigue, abdominal distension and belly aches, and even in some cases, behavior changes. The diagnosis of celiac disease is made by specific blood work that your doctor orders, in addition to a procedure called an endoscopy, which is only performed by an experienced pediatric gastroenterologist. Today, the endoscopy is still considered the gold standard for making the diagnosis for celiac disease in children, and a gluten-free diet remains the only treatment.

Without celiac disease (or a true food allergy to wheat), there is no real evidence-based indication for eliminating gluten from the diet. In fact, toddlers need carbohydrates from wheat, barley, and oats on a regular basis to supply B vitamins and adequate calories. From a health-care practitioner's perspective, it's hard to watch parents unnecessarily restrict an entire food group from their growing toddler's diet, especially if that toddler has struggled to gain weight. In addition, if you are concerned that your toddler is showing some warning signs of celiac and want to have him tested, he will need to be eating gluten in order for any of the tests and procedures to be reliable. Seek help from a pediatric gastroenterologist who specializes in treating digestive diseases (www.naspgn.org).

Constipation can be alleviated without completely cutting out gluten if you cut back on the refined grains in your household, such as white bread, sugary cereals, and other products made with "enriched white flour." Even though the labels say "white flour," it still contains gluten, as all white flours are whole-grain derived.

You can also try alternating grains: using brown rice and quinoa frequently are two good examples of how to approach this. In a sense, if you are alternating grains, you are offering your toddler a lower-gluten diet, which might make you feel a little better.

DIARRHEA

As we have already discussed chronic nonspecific diarrhea of toddlerhood (CNSD), I wanted to touch on acute diarrhea—as in the result of a virus, more commonly known as a stomach bug. It happens so frequently in this young population because so many toddlers spend a significant amount of time in a day-care setting and their immune systems are still immature. Parents get really worried about diarrhea that goes on for a week, and even more worried about what to (or what not to!) feed their toddler during these trying times. Acute diarrhea can be a disruption to potty training for sure in this age group, and parents often find themselves manipulating their toddler's diet to halt diarrhea in its tracks. If you have seen your pediatrician and she has ruled out any red flags that could indicate the diarrhea is being caused by something more serious, then read on for further advice.

Although this may seem illogical, it is entirely necessary to feed your toddler proper foods through the virus. During periods of acute diarrhea caused by a stomach bug, the small intestine, which is the organ responsible for absorbing nutrients from food, will benefit from nutritious foods to replenish and restore overall function. In essence, your toddler's "gut" needs to be nourished—not just him.

It is natural for your toddler to eat a lot less during times of a stomach virus—don't fret: he will make up the calories when he feels better. The most important thing to do is make sure he stays hydrated, and offer him small amounts of food regularly. If you ever have concerns about dehydration, prolonged periods of diarrhea, or see blood in your toddler's stool, call your pediatrician immediately.

For years, the most common diet parents subscribe to during bouts of diarrhea is called the BRAT diet, and some pediatricians are still recommending it. The BRAT diet stands for bananas, rice, applesauce, and tea or toast. This diet has been around for many years and used to be prescribed to help bind very loose stools. While it is fine to offer your toddler these foods for a day or two at the most, it is unsafe to continue the diet for an extended period of time. The BRAT diet lacks protein, sodium, calcium, phosphorus, and zinc—all of which are critical to helping a toddler get back on his feet, stay nourished, and grow.

What can we learn from the BRAT diet?

As some foods are clearly more binding than others, we can include these foods in our toddlers' diets to help thicken loose poop, with hopes to make the situation better, not worse. It should be noted that the foods in the BRAT diet are not binding when they are included as a part of a balanced diet, so there is no need to avoid giving them on a regular basis to toddlers who might be constipated. Read below for some suggestions as to what to offer your toddler with acute diarrhea.

Think starchy carbs with a touch of salt

When most people hear "salt," the words "avoid" and "high blood pressure" immediately run through their minds. When kids have diarrhea for a week or so, their bodies lose salt, which is an important mineral to maintain cell function and hydration status. You don't need to worry about salt during this time, and truth be told, small amounts of salt used in cooking for a family can be safe and necessary when feeding a toddler—especially when it comes to amplifying taste.

Here is a list of foods to offer your toddler when he has acute diarrhea or when his tummy hurts. Consider this your "sick" feeding plan:

- Whole wheat toast, English muffin, or mini bagel with one teaspoon butter
- Baked sweet or white potato (no skin) with one to two teaspoons butter and salt
- Chicken broth, with soft-cooked soup noodles and small carrots

- Oven-roasted chicken or turkey with brown rice (cook brown rice in chicken broth for an extra kick of salt, which is always needed during periods of rehydration)
- Egg noodles tossed in olive oil and salt
- Cream of wheat or oatmeal flavored with maple syrup or brown sugar
- Small amounts of yogurt smoothies to REAP the benefits of good bacteria
- A small amount of good frozen yogurt as a treat
- Applesauces; bananas; soft, small diced peaches; and even baked apples with a dash of cinnamon
- Sweet breads, such as pumpkin or banana
- Crunchy, salty snacks are well accepted and can provide extra calories and salt:
  - Pretzel Stix, Veggie Stix, Nude Food, potato chips (plain), Ritz crackers, saltines, or plain butter crackers
  - Dried fortified cereals can provide extra vitamins and minerals

What foods to avoid:

- Excess fruit juice consumption: while small sips of juice are fine during acute diarrhea, it is not wise to offer more than four ounces of juice during this time. Fruit juice has a lot of sugar in it, without any salt or potassium, so it can actually make diarrhea worse.

Avoid apple juice or apple juice blends, and stick with diluted cranberry, pomegranate, or white grape juice.

- Greasy, fried foods, especially fast food
- Excessive gas-producing foods: raw veggies, beans, broccoli, cauliflower
- Too much vitamin C—especially from a supplement. Vitamin C can be irritating to the GI tract; stick with fortified applesauces and packed fruits in juices for the time being.
- Excess berries or dried fruits: we have learned so far that these foods are super-high in insoluble fiber, which as a reminder is the kind of fiber that helps *increase* transit time in your small intestine—meaning foods move faster. In cases of diarrhea, we definitely do not want things moving faster through your toddler's GI tract!

The key is to be sure that you offer small portions of food every two to three hours and keep up with his fluid intake: Jell-O and Popsicles can help, but be sure to avoid sugar-free varieties as they contain artificial sweeteners that could make diarrhea worse.

What to drink

Milk: I frequently find that parents will stop giving their toddler milk during an acute viral illness, as many fear that the milk itself will make the problem worse. Don't withhold milk from a toddler who is asking for it—even with diarrhea. If you have seen your pediatrician, and your toddler has been given the diagnosis of stomach virus, drinking milk will not harm him—in fact, milk will provide key nutrients during a period where eating will not.

In some cases where diarrhea continues for up to two weeks, you might find your toddler poops less frequently while taking out milk from his diet. This can be true, as the sugar in milk (known as lactose) can be temporarily malabsorbed in a person who has been sick with a viral illness and diarrhea for two weeks or more.

If you find that milk seems to be aggravating your toddler, try switching for the duration of the virus to a lactose-free milk, which is available in your grocery store where regular milk is sold. Lactose-free milk provides all of the essential nutrients such as protein, fat, vitamins A and D, and calcium that regular milk provides, without the lactose. These milks are treated with an enzyme so that the lactose is already broken down before it hits your toddler's tummy. Once your toddler is feeling better, gradually try to introduce regular milk back into his diet by mixing it with regular milk (half lactose-free, half regular), then ultimately transition back to regular whole milk.

The goal is to get your toddler back on track with what he normally eats as soon as possible, and avoid unnecessary restrictions of foods that could limit his intake of vital nutrients for growth and development.

Water: We all know that water is the essence to staying hydrated. With toddlers who are experiencing diarrhea, drinking more water than usual with some food intake is generally fine and expected. Try offering shaved ice chips (not cubes, as they pose a choking hazard) for older toddlers to crunch on if they can only bear to take small sips. As you will read below, it is usually preferable to have your toddler sip on medically formulated rehydration solutions in addition to water during periods of acute dehydration.

Oral rehydration solutions (ORS): Oral rehydration solutions are designed to provide the small intestine with some sugar, salt, and potassium to help replenish electrolyte losses such as in cases of prolonged diarrhea and even vomiting. ORS have a lower sugar content than most sports drinks and are found in different varieties, such as Popsicles, and different flavors. Again, these solutions are devoid of calcium and other minerals, so they should not be used for extended periods of time in place of milk or milk equivalents. The most common ORS found at your local drug store is Pedialyte.

Sports drinks: Many parents tell me that their toddler refuses Pedialyte but will happily take Gatorade. This is not surprising, as most sports drinks will have more sugar than an ORS and overall less salt, so they tend to taste much better. For the record: sports drinks are not health food. Use caution when offering sports drinks to toddlers during periods of sickness if their diarrhea is not improving. I say it's best to mix the drink with an ORS and try to use a sports drink that has a lower sugar content. If your toddler is sipping on these drinks all day, she might want to have some every day, even when she is not sick. Take the time to casually explain to her that these drinks are for when her tummy doesn't feel so great—they are not an everyday choice. And be sure to check the label for any added herbals, protein, or high doses of vitamins—all of which are unnecessary and potentially unsafe for the toddler.

Diluted caffeine-free tea: Black teas can offer a punch of antioxidants, which are important for your immune system—even a tiny toddler's. For older toddlers, say two and three, sipping on diluted tea mixed with a small amount of honey and lemon can help them feel better and soothe their GI tract. Caveat: tea should never replace milk in a toddler's diet—even if you are adding milk to tea, it doesn't count, because tea contains tannic acid, which, when taken in large amounts, can interfere with calcium and even iron absorption.

DIGESTIVE SUPPLEMENTS TO CONSIDER

When toddlers suffer from a viral illness that affects their GI tract or have diarrhea associated with a course of antibiotics, many pediatricians and specialists might suggest starting a "probiotic supplement." As mentioned before, probiotics are health-promoting bacteria. Our GI tract contains billions of bugs that need to be kept in good balance—when your toddler gets sick or requires a course of antibiotics, the good bacteria that naturally live there can be depleted. And in order for ideal function, good bacteria need to be restored as soon as possible. This can be done by eating yogurt or kefir, which naturally contains live active cultures. Otherwise, a supplemental course can be given for a defined time period of about two to three weeks, and then discontinued.

By no means is this list of recommended probiotics and supplements exhaustive. However, the probiotics listed here have been studied the most and are easy to find online or at your local pharmacy. Some things to account for before starting any probiotic supplement:

- Check if your supplement requires refrigeration.
- Talk to your pediatrician before starting a probiotic if your toddler is immunocompromised in any way, or if he is on medication that suppresses his immune system.
- Mind the expiration date on the package, and be sure to toss once the product is expired.
- Do not give your toddler any antidiarrheal medication during periods of acute diarrhea, unless prescribed by your pediatrician. Diarrhea caused by a

virus is the body's natural defense mechanism for evacuating an unwanted interloper, so stopping the process with meds is not the best idea.

Culturelle Kids!: This probiotic perhaps has the most product recognition and can be purchased at your local pharmacies and grocery stores. Culturelle Kids! is milk-free and contains *Lactobacillus* GG, which is one of the most studied probiotics in the world. Use as directed on the package insert for up to three weeks. (www.culturelle.com)

BioGaia ProTectis: Developed and made in Sweden, this probiotic comes in a variety of forms which can help with compliance. Chewables, straws, and drops are some of the ways your toddler can take this product made with *Lactobacillus reuteri*. Follow the instructions on the package for dosing and administration. (www.biogaia.com)

Florastor Kids: This product is unique in that it is not a live bacteria but rather a safe strain of yeast that works to restore the flora of the intestine that might be weakened from illnesses such as diarrhea. This product, which contains *Saccharomyces boulardii*, does not stay in the digestive system, but rather passes through in about two to three days. Follow the instructions on the package for dosing and administration. (www.florastor.com)

Nana Flakes: Although it is not a probiotic, this product is a supplement that can be given for periods of acute diarrhea or ongoing nonspecific diarrhea of toddlerhood. Nana Flakes are dried bananas, which come in sachets (or very small pouches) and are a good source of pectin, a super soluble fiber that can bind loose stools to make them a bit more formed and easier to manage. Typical dosing is to add one packet to applesauce or milk up to three times per day. (www.nutritionaldesignsinc.com)

WHAT ELSE ABOUT DIGESTIVE HEALTH? THE SOAP BOX

So far, we have talked about the most common digestive challenges toddlers may face at some point between years one and three—and unfortunately, even beyond. You might be wondering what else you can do to optimize your toddler's digestion, even if he doesn't suffer from chronic constipation or bouts of diarrhea. The best advice I can give, and one that I find proves tried and true time and time again, is (drum roll, please) home-cooked meals. I know, the answer is at best underwhelming and possibly even frustrating.

More home-cooked meals simply means less processed foods, and less processed foods means better digestive health.

Don't panic. There are *so many* decent convenience foods available out there that homemade can easily be translated into semi-homemade. That being said, taking time to learn some simple healthy recipes that put "homemade" food on your table at least three to four nights per week is a reasonable and attainable goal to achieve. Here are some tips to get you started:

1. Shop on Saturdays and cook on Sundays. Weekend planning is essential for a few meals that are homemade. Shopping on Saturday and cooking something on Sunday will help you start the week off right.

2. Plan for vegetables. Rely on fresh and frozen vegetables, and be sure to cook them with intention. So often people will pour a bag of frozen green beans into boiling water and call it a side dish. Amplify with flavor and add a touch of salt, pepper, garlic, and even some oil or butter to make them taste yummy.

3. Simplify your side dishes. Don't rely only on boxes of highly processed rice, instant potatoes, or pasta products. Make your own flavorful sides by starting with the food in its most natural state and then adding seasonings on your own to amplify the flavor.

4. Subscribe to cooking blogs, "family" food websites, and sign up for email blasts from the ones you find you

rely on the most. I personally love simplyrecipes.com, epicurious.com, and wholefoods.com.

5. Refer back to chapter six for staple recipes of popular toddler meals that you can learn to prepare with a healthier twist.

CHAPTER EIGHT

The Family Table

Hopefully you have now learned that much of eating and feeding is not just about the food we put in front of our kids. More so, it is the approach to feeding. Take a few minutes to recall the main ideas presented so far that will foster healthy eating habits for years to come:

- Where your toddler sits to eat
- Who eats with him
- Maintaining an established routine of scheduled meals and snacks

We have also learned three key concepts that apply to mealtime:

- Introducing a new food
- Continuously exposing your toddler to foods
- Expanding the food choices

We can go one last step further and recap the ground rules for mealtime.

THE FAMILY TABLE: IF YOU BUILD IT, THEY WILL COME

The most important action you can do for your toddler to support her eating habits is build your family table. I don't mean go out and bang some nails together to make a homemade version of what you might find on sale at Pottery Barn (that would be scary). Building a family table simply means setting your expectations and ground rules for mealtimes and beginning to teach them to your toddler as early as one year of age. Take a look at this example.

Jane's Story

Jane was a patient who came to me for counseling on slow weight gain and "picky eating." She was turning three in the next few months, and both of her parents accompanied her to the visit. The chief concern her father had was that she could never just "eat" what her mother made for dinner that night like her other siblings did. Jane would whine and cry and shove her plate away, and then her mom would get up from the table and make her something different. Essentially, Jane's mother was acting like a short-order cook. This action then disrupted the whole family dinner, because the other kids would start questioning why Jane got such special attention and why they too couldn't have their favorite food night after night. What made it worse was when Jane barely ate what her mom had personally made just for her.

As I sat and listened to their story, it was obvious that Jane's parents felt pretty bad about the whole situation—they just couldn't figure out how to fix it. When I asked them what their ground rules were for the dinner table, they both gave me a respectable list of table manners:

- They wash their hands before dinner.
- They say grace before dinner.
- They say "excuse me" if they burp.
- They say "please" and "thank you" when passing serving bowls.
- They drink milk or water with meals (no soda allowed).
- They ask if they may be excused before leaving.
- The older kids bring their dishes to the sink.

Truth be told, I was quite impressed. When I asked Jane's parents how their children knew to do these things, her mom simply stated, "Because those are the rules." With that one sentence, I knew I could provide a solution—I just had to sell it.

After applauding both parents for having structured mealtimes and instilling admirable table manners in their kids, I asked them if they felt there was room for one more "rule" they could apply to dinnertime: *no short-order cooking allowed.*

At first, Jane's mom looked confused, but then I went on to explain: the rules are the rules, right? Jane was young enough to buy into this concept, as she was already following most of the rules they had told me about. I told her parents the next time Jane refused to eat what the family was eating and demanded something different, they should just tell her that she could eat something from the table that was being served, just like everybody else. That was the rule, plain and simple.

We went on to discuss some counter-strategies to Jane's expected protests, and I assured the parents that this would take time, so everyone needed to be patient. I talked with them about using a safety food and being totally calm and neutral in their response to her outburst. The goal was to eventually make the situation better, not worse. Over time, Jane would learn to come to the table and eat what her mother made for dinner, and she would probably start to gain weight a bit better, once she learned to like some new foods.

After several months, I did get a phone call from Jane's dad, surprisingly. He explained that since we met, they made a point to practice this each night at dinner. At first it was difficult, but over time, Jane started catching on to the new rule. Jane's dad explained that her *siblings* were in part responsible for the big success. Whenever something was put on the table that Jane didn't like, they all encouraged her to be like them and follow the rules.

Jane's story is a perfect example of "if you build it, they will come." Set your expectations and uphold them—toddlers thrive on structure and routine and will grow up feeling secure and confident while looking forward to coming to the table, simply because they know what to expect.

GROUND RULES FOR MEALTIME

As parents, we never want our kids to dread coming to the dinner table. Dinnertime is not the place to debate about who has more to do, how miserable your boss might be, or how poorly one of your kids might be doing in school. Take a look below at some more basic rules that will help mealtime be successful.

Don't become a short-order cook. As we heard in Jane's story, short-order cooking can disrupt mealtime and allows your toddler to have all the control in deciding what he wants to eat; kids will never learn to like new foods if they are not challenged to do so. Short-order cooking is one of the biggest causes of "picky eating" and probably one of the most overlooked by parents and health-care professionals. Make it a rule in your house that your toddler finds something to eat on the table. It might just be the corn you serve that night with a few spoons of rice and bite of bread—so be it.

The long-term consequences of being catered to are far worse than the short-term consequences of one nutritionally inferior meal a few times a week.

Modify meals to help the toddler succeed. In short, don't serve foods they just can't manage. You don't have to be a martyr when it comes to making family meals. Under no condition would I expect you to serve your toddler a piece of steak that wasn't cut up into small manageable pieces. Nor would I expect you to serve your toddler who clearly doesn't like hot food spicy Thai chicken with peanut sauce simply because that is "what's for dinner." Instead, learn to make "grown-up" foods kid-friendly by altering the *flavor* if needed—not the entire meal. Take the spicy Thai chicken example: set a piece of the plain cooked chicken aside before adding heat to the whole dish; dice it up into small pieces and then toss lightly in a mixture of one teaspoon of mild peanut sauce, one teaspoon of canola oil, and a touch of honey. Serve the chicken with the same rice and veggies, and voila! In minutes, you essentially have the same meal for your tot that the rest of the family is eating—without making the toddler "separate food."

Be open to the early-bird special. There is no doubt that dinnertime is the most difficult meal of the day for the one- to three-year-old. Parents incessantly comment on how they can't stand dinnertime because their toddler is just so cranky. Ultimately, this leads to doling out a snack before dinner that ends up being the perfect amount of food to spoil it altogether. The best solution to this is to eat earlier if possible. If you find your toddler is looking for snacks and on the verge of a complete meltdown around 4:45, then let dinner begin. As a dietitian, I would rather have you feed your toddler proper food at 4:45 than have her eat some pretzels and then forgo the nutritious main meal at 5:30. Typically, once toddlers reach the age of three, they can manage waiting to sit down to dinner by 5:30 or 6:00 p.m.

Sit together. By sitting together for family dinners, you can not only be a good role model for your toddler when it comes to healthy eating, but you can also show your toddler that he is part of a family—which is especially important for such an egocentric age. Toddlers can learn table manners, practice waiting their turn to speak, and even learn to enjoy sharing their favorite part of the day. The routine of family dinner has also been shown to decrease the prevalence of obesity in U.S. preschool-age children by 40 percent.

Be consistent when setting boundaries at the table. So many parents of picky eaters feel completely disarmed when they see their tot blatantly refusing to eat. Some parents may resort to punishing the toddler on some nights, bribing on another night, or even making her new food on yet another night just to get her to eat *something*. I too have felt the frustrations so many parents tell me about, and while this reaction is understandable, it is also the worst-case scenario for the picky eater. Make it a rule for yourself to handle her eating (or lack of) consistently each night. Go back to some of the suggestions in the beginning of the book for staying calm and firm when mealtime doesn't go exactly as planned:

1. Start small! Present food in small portions and in manageable pieces.

2. Ignore the "I'm done!" remark by redirecting conversation.

3. Resist the urge to bribe or beg your child to just take one more bite.

4. Always remember that toddlers can have a knee-jerk reaction when being presented with new food and say "I don't like that!" just because it's something unfamiliar. Give them the chance to take a risk and try the new food on their own before you try to solve it for them and serve them something differ- ent. (Yes, helicopter parenting applies to eating.)

5. Put an end to pan-handling. If your toddler hops down from the table, the meal is over. Gently remind

him of that before he gets down by calmly saying, "Are you sure you are finished? I just don't want you to be hungry again before bath time." Make sure if you go out on a limb to say this that you stick to your guns when he comes back in five minutes for a few more bites of food. Say, "Dinner is over when you get down from the table."

6. Remove your toddler from the table if she becomes unruly. This doesn't have to be dramatic—although consider yourself forewarned that it usually ends up that way. If your toddler is miserable and disrupting dinnertime for everyone else, then she needs to be removed from the situation altogether and given a chance to calm down. I know: who wants to deal with a time-out at dinnertime? You are probably tired and hungry and just want to sit down and eat in peace. But you wouldn't let your toddler act unruly at a play-date or birthday party, right? Mealtime is the same. Teach her early that the family table is no place to throw a fit.

Keep in mind again that dinnertime can be so hard for toddlers because they are just too tired (so if you are wondering if you should be putting your feisty three-year-old who no longer naps in a time-out when dinner is at 6:30 each night, think again and try eating earlier!).

WHAT ELSE CAN WE LEARN? A WORD ON THE EPIDEMIC OF PEDIATRIC OBESITY

I truly believe much of the confusion surrounding feeding toddlers and children stems from the fear of raising an obese child. Statistics from the Centers for Disease Control and Prevention tell us that 17 percent of U.S. children ages two to nineteen are obese, with the prevalence of obesity tripling since the eighties. It seems like simple math really, when you consider what has happened to our portions of food. What parents may not know is that this "epidemic" is not created equal and is considerably complex. Some groups of people are affected more seriously than others, with factors such as ethnicity, age, socioeconomic status, and even where you live in the United States, all contributing to the prevalence of pediatric obesity.

It is obvious there is an alarmingly high number of children and adolescents today who are extremely overweight; I see many of them in our liver clinic each month.

However, for the children who are not plotting above the 95th percentile in their weight for age alone or jumping off the growth curve in the course of six months to a year, the problem may be that they are awaiting natural linear growth, particularly the toddler.

Body mass index (BMI), which has become a regular tool in the pediatrician's office for assessing weight and obesity, has its limits—especially for the young toddler. The cut-off points to define when a child is given the diagnosis of "obese" were subjectively appointed based on what children were weighing in at a few decades ago, with complete neglect for current health statistics, not to mention that many toddlers will gain body weight before they actually get taller, leaving them with the potential on paper to appear "short and fat" at any given office visit. In addition, some people (including toddlers) simply are built more solidly than others due to genetic makeup. The best example of this is the athlete: many people with an athletic build have more muscle mass, and muscle weighs more than fat; therefore, they weigh more. Lastly, food is not entirely responsible for obesity—actually, it's really just a piece of the puzzle, with lack of physical activity, inadequate nighttime sleep, and fewer home-cooked meals being big contributing factors as well.

For many of you with a picky eater, raising an overweight child might not be of utmost concern; right now, your focus is most likely on whether or not he eats at all. However, in my practice from time to time, we meet parents of picky eaters whose issues have resolved, and they are happily eating just about everything. To my surprise, during the course of a follow-up visit, some of these parents are now overly concerned about their toddler becoming too heavy, when just months ago they were barely gaining weight. With further conversation, I often begin to understand that this idea of becoming "overweight" or getting "too heavy" was often a seed planted by a well-intended family doctor.

Here are some things you need to know if your toddler has been given a "warning" about becoming overweight, or worse been called obese right in the office.

1. Ask your toddler's doctor to see her growth chart, so you can have a better understanding of the trend and velocity of her growth—both in height and weight and not just the calculated BMI. If your toddler appears proportional and is growing at a higher percentile curve for both weight and height, don't panic—she might just end up being "bigger." Or, if her weight percentile is higher than her height percentile, give her some time to catch up and stick to your plan of regularly scheduled meals and snacks with a modest increase in activity. Healthy people come in all shapes and sizes, and for girls, most importantly, body acceptance needs to start from day one. At all costs, parents should avoid commenting on their child's body size, because he will feel like something is wrong with him or, even worse, that they are not happy with who he is. Children have the right to feel that love is not conditional on frame size or body weight.

2. If your pediatrician made the grave mistake of talking about *weight loss* in front of your tot or using the term "overweight and/or obese," you as the parent need to undo that lingo and reframe it in a positive light. Words need to be changed to support a positive intent with the focus on overall health, not weight. For example, you can say, "OK, Amy, it sounds like we should get outside and ride our bikes together to keep our hearts healthy and build strong muscles. Spike [the family dog] will be so excited to take an extra spin around the block with us at night."

3. Take the focus away from food. As mentioned above, food is just a piece of the puzzle to pediatric obesity. Today, our children are eating a diet that is low in nutrients and high in empty calories. That, in short, is a recipe for excess body weight, not to mention poor digestive function. For the toddler, this is of utmost importance, as early introduction to proper food (nutrient-rich food) can set the stage for a lifetime of good eating habits. Instead of resorting to food restriction, which is beyond miserable for everyone involved—and dangerous for the toddler—increase activity, decrease television viewing time, and say no to handheld gaming systems for kids under six years old.

4. One of the strongest childhood predictors of becoming obese as an adult is having an obese parent, so take your own weight seriously. This does not mean start weighing yourself every day or begin a fad diet that will leave you deprived and craving food. In fact, experts on eating disorders say you should never talk about your body weight or size in front of your kids because they will internalize the message that it is your physical appearance that matters most. Instead, be a good role model and make healthy food choices on most days, be comfortable eating less than perfectly on others, exercise regularly, and have a positive body image of yourself. Your toddler came from that body, and by the time he is four, he knows it!

5. Remember that the regulation of appetite and portion distortion begins as early as late infancy through toddlerhood. I cringe at the sight of the mother at the park, working tirelessly to get her toddler to eat every last bite of a fast-food kiddie meal; however, I also cringe at the mother who is bribing her three-year-old to finish every last bite of his turkey and cheese sandwich on two slices of whole-wheat bread. Both of these situations are examples of well-intended parents forcing food into their tot, never allowing her to reap the benefits of satiety—the biggest defense against the war on obesity.

A recent study published from the AAP showed that regular exposure to three household routines decreased the prevalence of obesity in U.S. preschool-age children (four-year-olds).

They were:

- eating the evening meal as a family more than five nights per week
- obtaining adequate nighttime sleep of at least 10.5 hours per night
- limiting screen viewing time to less than two hours per day on weekdays

SPECIAL CIRCUMSTANCES: EATING AT CELEBRATIONS AND HOLIDAYS

To me, there is nothing better than sitting down together and sharing a meal—especially at the holidays. However, it can be all too easy for food battles to creep their way into the dining room during a special celebration, inevitably causing unnecessary stress for the parents and the toddler.

The best advice I give to parents for handling holiday dinners or celebrations is simple: let it go. This can sometimes be difficult, particularly if Aunt Jean comments over and over again at how little food your little Johnny eats! In most cases, snacks and appetizers have been eaten before dinnertime, so many toddlers really won't be motivated to come sit down for a traditional roast and vegetables. Holidays are not the time or place to be worried about what or how much food your toddler ate or didn't. The most important thing about family holiday dinners is being together and establishing a tradition. Keep in mind these simple strategies to manage holiday meals:

1. Lower your expectations. Put just one or two tablespoons of two foods being served on your toddler's plate.

2. Allow her to have as much bread as she likes—it might keep her seated longer.

3. Talk to older toddlers ahead of mealtime. You can express to your three-year-old that it's important to sit together and be polite while he is seated at the dinner table.

4. Set a kids' table. Little ones can feel included and special that they have their own table to sit at. Quite honestly, *I* still love sitting at the kids' table. In our big extended family, you can be sure to find my husband or myself holding court at the kids' table, listening to their stories and encouraging conversations. Just by sitting with them, you are showing toddlers that they too are an important part of the

family. Make it festive and fun by putting a special treat on each child's seat, such as a chocolate gold coin or a special holiday drinking cup and straw at each place setting. For a real crowd pleaser, have their names written on them!

KEEP THE PEACE IN YOUR HOME: TAKE THE FOCUS OFF THE FOOD

From time to time, you will feel like you are at your wits end when trying to feed a picky toddler. Don't give up! Let it go for two weeks and take the focus away from *actual* food. Instead, try and channel your energy into exposing your toddler to the *concept* of food with these subliminal activities that shine a positive light on eating and make food actually seem fun.

Playing with food

Sometimes, you may need a break from feeling like you are trying so hard to get your little one to eat. Believe it or not, there are many ways to get your toddler thinking about food and eating in a positive way and have some fun at the same time. Many parents find that "food play" takes away the pressure that can accompany actual eating.

- Imaginary play: Use a play kitchen and toy food (plastic or wood) to allow your toddler to make her own dinners while you are cooking. Make sure to talk with her about what she is making and ask her to share what she cooks. This kind of imaginary play won't necessarily make her come to the table and gobble up her meal; however, it serves as positive reinforcement surrounding food, and might just make her a bit more interested in eating.

- Set up a "restaurant" or a grocery store aisle in your playroom, where you can line up different empty boxes of packaged foods or put play food on shelves. If you have a basket or a toy shopping cart, she can have fun filling one up and then checking out. Talking with her about what she bought is a great way to encourage her to try a new food. For example, if she has a play pear in her bag, you can say something like "Look Martha, I bought a pear today too (show her a real pear). Let's slice it up and see how good it is."

Read about food

There are many children's books that have food as the subject. Reading to your toddler is something you probably already do on a regular basis. Seek out stories where food is involved and take time going through the pictures. I often find it useful to read a book about food and then to make that food, being sure to remind him about the story. This engages a toddler's curiosity and he really seems to find it quite funny. So the next time you read Laura Numeroff's *If You Give a Pig a Pancake*, be sure to have a box of Bisquick on hand for the following morning—or try the from-scratch recipe listed in chapter six. You can reread the story before you make the pancakes—but be sure to let him stir the batter!

Other books on food:

Cloudy with a Chance of Meatballs, Judi Barrett
If You Give a Moose a Muffin, Laura Numeroff
Chicken Soup with Rice, Maurice Sendak
The Little Red Hen (Makes a Pizza), Philemon Sturges
Strega Nona, Tomie dePaola
The Very Hungry Caterpillar, Eric Carle
Bread and Jam for Frances, Russell Hoban
Spot Bakes a Cake, Eric Hill
Pickin' Peas, Margaret Read MacDonald
Gus and Button, Saxton Freymann
Green Eggs and Ham, Dr. Seuss
Blueberries for Sal, Robert McCloskey
James and the Giant Peach, Roald Dahl
The Giant Jam Sandwich, John Vernon Lord and
    Janet Burroway
How Do Dinosaurs Eat Their Food? Jane Yolen
First Book of Sushi, Amy Wilson Sanger
Mangia! Mangia! Amy Wilson Sanger
A Little Bit of Soul Food, Amy Wilson Sanger
Let's Nosh! Amy Wilson Sanger

Listen to music about food

Kids love music. Seek out CDs that include songs about food, and pop them in the car for long drives—or even short trips around town. Make sure you say things like, "Oh, we should try 'The Pretzel Store'" by Laurie Berkner or see how quickly they start singing "Fruit Salad (Yummy Yummy)" by the Wiggles. Then, when you are home, you can say, "It's time to make yummy, yummy fruit salad like the Wiggles!"

Other good food songs:

That's Amore, Dean Martin
Salad Groove and other songs on Joy Bauer's CD for kids
Albuquerque Turkey
Apples and Bananas
Apples in Pajamas
On Top of Spaghetti...
The Muffin Man
Vegetable Soup, the Wiggles
Go Bananas, Fresh Beat Band

Watch TV with awareness

We all know how commercials seep into the subconscious of kids and make them beg for the featured products at the store. I'll never forget the time when my son Jake at age six asked me why we couldn't buy Fruity Pebbles. He put up a solid argument by saying: "On the commercial they said it was a complete breakfast"! If your toddler has a favorite character on TV, use it to your advantage. Many characters talk about food and your toddler will notice. I am not claiming that your toddler will run into the kitchen and say, "Mom! Periwinkle from *Blues Clues* had waffles for breakfast—I want waffles." But she might get the idea and ask at some point. What you can do is be aware of what characters on the shows she watches are eating and *ask* her if she wants to have waffles like Periwinkle.

Cook with your toddlers

Some of the best childhood memories I have are when my parents were cooking on a Friday night—my dad was such an influence in the kitchen from as early as I can remember, and his specialty when I was younger was making homemade pasta. He invested in this pasta machine, and he would crank up Steve Winwood (now I am really dating myself!) and let us help. It was a way to spend time together. Obviously I was much older than a toddler when this was happening, but cooking with a toddler can be fun—as long as you are prepared and organized. Simple tasks like measuring flour, laying cheese on bread, blending fruit in a smoothie (with supervision), and stirring are all things toddlers can and want to do. If your toddler is motivated by imaginary play, he might even want to use an apron or a chef's hat. I highly recommend buying a Learning Tower, which will allow your child to get to counter level safely without standing on a chair or stool (www.littlepartners .com) so that your child can fully (and safely) work with you in the kitchen. Be prepared for messes, and be sure to be patient with your little toddler's learning curve.

Eat with friends

Parents often tell me their toddlers eat well at school—maybe it's the little table and chairs that are so inviting—but their eating is influenced by the fact that those around them are eating. Nothing leads to feeding success like peer pressure. This can take time for many older toddlers who might be new to a preschool setting, so be patient if you feel your toddler is not eating well at school, even with friends. I am a firm believer that starting a traditional day for "family dinner" or what many refer to as Sunday dinner is an important experience for toddlers. Having extended family or friends eat together can work just as well as having kids eat together at preschool. Some good websites I often refer to in order to reinforce why eating together is so important:

www.dinnertogether.com
www.raisinghappiness.com
www.ellynsatter.com

www.chopchopmag.org
www.thefamilydinnerbook.com

WHEN ALL ELSE FAILS...

If you are still feeling frustrations, even after reading this book, and your toddler just can't seem to "give peas a chance," then take a few minutes to decide what exactly your feeding goals are for your toddler. Write them down, and then ask yourself if they are realistic. If not, take a moment to refocus your goals.

Goal #1: I want my toddler to eat green vegetables every day.

Goal #1 reframed: I would like to see my toddler try to eat green vegetables three times per week at dinner.

The second goal is obviously much more realistic, considering all that we have just learned about how toddler eating habits can vary so vastly. The reframed goal allows you to be flexible with what your tot chooses to eat, which is in essence the most important thing you can do to support your child's eating habits, and raise a happy and confident eater.

Goal #2: I won't comment on my toddler's expression of dislikes of any particular food.

Goal #2 reframed: When my toddler doesn't like a particular food, I will say something positive such as "That's OK. Maybe you might like spinach when you're a little older. Everybody is different." Just remember to keep offering that food moving forward!

Goal #3: I want my toddler to only eat meals sitting at the table.

Goal #3 reframed: As a family, we will only eat food when we are sitting at the table.

This goal is actually a very realistic application to shoot for, but be sure to apply it to everyone in your family so your toddler follows suit and feels like part of the herd. Obvious exceptions to this rule are popcorn or the equivalent for family movie night or Popsicles on the front step after a visit from the ice cream truck.

For more on picky eating at every age, read about the registry that Duke University researchers have started. The registry can be found online at www .dukehealth.org/services/ eating_disorders/about. On the right side of the page, click on the Finicky Eating in Adults study link.

Goal #4: I want my toddler to learn to eat sandwiches for lunch, so I can pack them for preschool this fall.

Goal #4 reframed: I will start introducing sandwiches at lunchtime a few times a week and know ahead of time that she may still take them apart. Developmentally, she might not like things "mixed together."

Keep a record of these goals, and see what happens over the next six months. Giving ample time to allow for success is key to reaching your goals. You might be surprised to find out how motivating these small successes can be.

Some kids might just be picky forever, and if that ends up happening to your toddler as he gets older, at least you know you tried your best. The early years are the most important for exposing to foods. Don't resign your toddler to being a picky eater by throwing in the towel and giving up on all attempts to make healthy food and expose him to new flavors. Instead, allow him to grow up feeling educated about nutritious food choices and let him know you are not going to bend over backward just to get him to eat.

WHAT STUDIES SHOW

After working with families of picky eaters, I often find myself justifying the interventions and suggestions with actual data. Most of the time, I think I feel compelled to justify why, as a health-care professional, there is not a simple solution to make a kid eat. Some families find it helpful to know there is a whole body of evidence out there supporting the recommendations that I seem to make with such ease. Believe me when I say that there is nothing easy about this struggle between a parent and a child, and research shows us this. So I share that with the families.

At the end of a session, I have said countless times to the families struggling with picky eating in their home, "This isn't me just making this stuff up. It's based on years of research supporting the direct connection between parenting and feeding."

Read some real excerpts from studies conducted by medical and behavioral researchers on picky eating and parental behaviors surrounding it.

Copy these sentences and stick them on your fridge for when you need them most. Living with a toddler, you might just need to read them every day.

- Results showed that pressure is only effective if it's done indirectly by modeling enjoyment while eating.
- When offering a new food, parents need to provide many more repeated exposures (e.g., eight to fifteen times) to enhance acceptance of that food than they currently do.
- Parents consuming more fruits and vegetables

were less likely to pressure their daughters to eat and had daughters who were less picky and consumed more fruits and vegetables.

- Picky eating is a common disorder during childhood often causing considerable parental anxiety.
- Picky eating is an aspect of child development. Children will develop their own preferences when given the appropriate tools to do so. Parents are their children's greatest role models.
- Parents create environments for children that may foster the development of healthy eating behaviors and weight, or that may contribute to weight problems and eating disorders. In conclusion, positive parental role models may be a better method for improving a child's diet than attempts at dietary control.

Resources

Ames, Louise Bates, and Frances L. Ilq. *Your One-Year-Old: The Fun Loving, Fussy 12- to 24-Month-Old.* New York: Dell Publishing, 1983.

———. *Your Three-Year-Old: Friend or Enemy.* New York: Dell Publishing, 1980.

———. *Your Two-Year-Old: Terrible or Tender.* New York: Dell Publishing, 1980.

Badger, T. M., et al. "The health implications of soy infant formula." *American Journal of Clinical Nutrition* 89 (suppl): 1668S–72S.

Bisanz, J. E. "Unraveling How Probiotic Yogurt Works." *Science Translational Medicine* 3 (2011), 41.

"Centers for Disease Control and Prevention." www.cdc.gov.

"Delish." www.delish.com.

"Dietary Reference Intakes," last modified September 19, 2012. http://fnic.nal.usda.gov/dietary-guidance/dietary-reference-intakes

"Dietary Supplement Fact Sheet: Calcium," last modified August 1, 2012. http://ods.od.nih.gov/factsheets/Calcium-HealthProfessional/

"Eat Right. Academy of Nutrition and Dietetics." www
.eatright.org.

"Eating Disorders." www.dukehealth.org/services/eating
_disorders/about.

Fletcher, Dr. Janice, and Dr. Laurel Branen. "Feeding
Young Children in Group Settings." University of
Idaho, Agricultural and Life Sciences.

Fox, M. K., et al. "Average portions of foods commonly
eaten by infants and toddlers in the United States."
Journal of the American Dietetic Association 106
(2006): S66–S76.

Greer, F. R., Sicherer S., et al. "Effects of Early
Nutritional Interventions on the Development of
Atopic Disease in Infants and Children: The Role
of Maternal Dietary Restriction, Breastfeeding,
Timing of Introduction of Complementary Foods."
Pediatrics 121 (2008), 183.

Klein, Marsha Dunn. "Tube Feeding Transition
Plateaus." *Exceptional Parent Magazine* 36 (6).

Kleinman, Ronald E., M.D., and American Academy
of Pediatrics Committee on Nutrition. *Pediatric
Nutrition Handbook, 5th Edition*. Elk Grove:
American Academy of Pediatrics, 2004.

"Kraft Foods." www.kraftfoodandfamily.com

Larson, N., et al. "What Role Can a Child Care Setting
Play in Obesity Prevention?" *Journal of the American
Dietetic Association* 111 (2011): 1343–1362.

Lowenburg, M. E. "Development of food patterns in young children." *Nutrition in Infancy and Childhood, fourth edition,* by Christine Marie Trahms and Peggy L. Pipes.

"Meal Makeover Moms." www.mealmakeovermoms .com.

Pollan, Michael. *In Defense of Food: An Eater's Manifesto.* New York: Penguin, 2009.

Samour, Pamela Queen, and Kathy King. *Handbook of Pediatric Nutrition, Third Edition.* Burlington: Jones and Bartlett Learning, 2005.

Satter, Ellyn. *Child of Mine: Feeding with Love and Good Sense.* Boulder: Bull Publishing, 2000.

———. *How to Get Your Kid to Eat... But Not Too Much.* Boulder: Bull Publishing, 1987.

"Simply Recipes." www.simplyrecipes.com.

"Super Healthy Kids." http://blog.superhealthykids .com.

"Tiny Tummies." www.tinytummies.com.

"USDA ChooseMyPlate.gov." www.choosemyplate .gov.

Wang, Yourfa. "Disparities in Pediatric Obesity in the United States." *Advances in Nutrition* 2 (2011): 23-21.

Wyllie, Robert, M.D., and Jeffrey S. Hyams, M.D. *Pediatric Gastrointestinal and Liver Disease, fourth edition.* Philadelphia: Saunders, 2011.

Acknowledgments

A wise person told me once when I was in college always to surround myself with quality people. This resonated with me, and today I sit here with a long list of people I am lucky enough to call my family, friends, colleagues, and confidants. These people seem to transcend into the highest rank of quality, if that is at all possible, and without them in my life, I am not sure this book could have or would have happened. First, I will forever be indebted to my friend Joy Bauer for giving me the opportunity to succeed in writing and always taking the time to provide clear thought and direction, despite her very hectic life.

My editors, Kelly Bale and Shana Drehs, at Sourcebooks, for keeping things moving and providing exceptional direction for a health-care professional writing her first book ever.

My agent Jessica Papin, for never giving up on *Peas* and providing positive support all the while, connecting me with Sheila Oakes, the editor who shaped the proposal that sold.

I feel so lucky to have moved back to Connecticut,

where I was fortunate enough to be hired by Dr. Jeffrey Hyams and Claire Dalidowicz to work with the picky population at Connecticut Children's Medical Center (CCMC) in the Division of Digestive Diseases, Hepatology, and Nutrition. *Give Peas a Chance* was born in suite 2K, and gratitude goes out to everyone there for all of their support, as well as the Department of Clinical Nutrition.

Special thanks goes out to my colleagues and friends at CCMC who regularly offered advice and opinions and answered unrelenting text messages—and even gave hugs without hesitation: Karan Emerick, MD; Beth Chatfield, RD; Lauren Arata, RD; Sue Goodine, RD; Petra Amrein, RN; and Joanne Arena, RD. In addition, I want to distinctively thank my good friend and colleague at CCMC, Kate Vance, RD, who saw me through this whole journey not only on a professional level by willingly brainstorming toddler meal plans over several lunch hours, but who also was a tremendous support on a personal level. Kate was always able to bring me back to the basic science of nutrition, which kept me focused and helped me to keep things simple and carry on.

To Renee and Amy, my sisters-in-law, and to my brother Chris, for always being there on my five-minute drive home from Starbucks when I needed to get an opinion on food—or just to vent and laugh about life with kids and lots of work to do.

For Nana and Pop-Pop, Victoria and the late William Tammone, for being the greatest cooks on Earth and giving me my most cherished childhood memories of food, family, and tradition.

My parents, Patsy and Tom Molnar, have been my number-one fans for as long as I can recall. Their genuine support for all I commit myself to is never-ending, and every day I am a parent myself, I realize how lucky I was, and still am, to have them as my mom and dad. Thanks for paving the way (and Patsy—for always cooking my family dinner in my absence).

To Jake and Maggie, my amazing kids, for teaching me every day to see life through the eyes of a child. You both gave me the insight to make this book happen!

Lastly, and most importantly, I want to thank my husband Brian. Not just for keeping our family routine in check every night as I zipped out the door to write: doing dishes, playing outside, giving baths, getting snacks, and reading bedtime stories my way; but more importantly, for always believing in my dreams, no matter what. Thanks, Coach.

About the Author

Kate Samela, MS, RD, CSP, has been a registered dietitian for twelve years and is board certified by the Commission on Dietetic Registration as a specialist in pediatric nutrition. After obtaining a master's degree in clinical nutrition from New York University, 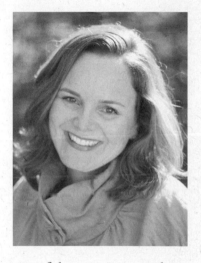 she spent the next ten years of her career working with children of all ages, prescribing nutrition therapy and counseling families on feeding and nutrition. She found a passion for teaching and has taught the topic of pediatric nutrition to hundreds of medical, nutrition, and nursing students throughout the east coast, at Mount Sinai Hospital in New York City, and as an adjunct professor at New York University College of Education, Hunter College in New York City, University of Connecticut, St. Joseph's College, and

Connecticut Children's Medical Center. During this time, she wrote several magazine articles on nutrition for *Big Apple Parent* and *Parent Magazine*, as well as a chapter appendix and an online teaching module for medical students for the American Society of Parenteral and Enteral Nutrition (ASPEN). She was the lead author for a research publication in the medical journal *Progress in Transplant*.

She has spoken on children's nutrition to audiences of all sizes, including the Greater New York Dietetic Association Annual Convention, Connecticut Organization of Neonatal Nurses Annual Conference, Connecticut Children's Medical Center Nursing Education and Development program, the American Dietetic Association, and the International Small Bowel Transplant Symposium.

Her extensive didactic and clinical training provided her with an advanced understanding of how little bodies grow and thrive. This set the foundation for transitioning to private counseling at one of the country's largest private practices, Joy Bauer Nutrition, where she counseled and designed food plans for young children and adolescents.

Currently, she works at Connecticut Children's Medical Center as an outpatient dietitian for the Division of Digestive Diseases, Hepatology, and Nutrition, which cares for over ten thousand patients per year. Here, she has been able to tie together her passion for the

nutritional management of digestive problems and poor growth and gets a firsthand opportunity to provide realistic nutrition advice to hundreds of families struggling with basic feeding issues for otherwise healthy toddlers.

She lives in Connecticut with her husband and two children—one of whom is still in the stage of picky eating!